PANDEMICS AND THE MEDIA

GLOBAL CRISES AND THE MEDIA

Simon Cottle
General Editor

Vol. 12

The Global Crises and the Media series is part
of the Peter Lang Media and Communication list.
Every volume is peer reviewed and meets
the highest quality standards for content and production.

PETER LANG
New York • Bern • Frankfurt • Berlin
Brussels • Vienna • Oxford • Warsaw

MARINA LEVINA

PANDEMICS AND THE MEDIA

PETER LANG
New York • Bern • Frankfurt • Berlin
Brussels • Vienna • Oxford • Warsaw

Library of Congress Cataloging-in-Publication Data

Levina, Marina.
Pandemics and the media / Marina Levina.
pages cm. — (Global crises and the media; vol. 12)
Includes bibliographical references and index.
1. AIDS (Disease) and mass media. 2. Epidemics—Press coverage.
3. Blood—Symbolic aspects. 4. Blood—Social aspects. I. Title.
P96.A39L863 362.1'042—dc23 2014024884
ISBN 978-1-4331-1552-3 (hardcover)
ISBN 978-1-4331-1551-6 (paperback)
ISBN 978-1-4539-1406-9 (e-book)
ISSN 1947-2587

Bibliographic information published by **Die Deutsche Nationalbibliothek**.
Die Deutsche Nationalbibliothek lists this publication in the "Deutsche Nationalbibliografie"; detailed bibliographic data are available on the Internet at http://dnb.d-nb.de/.

29 Broadway, 18th floor, New York, NY 10006
www.peterlang.com

For my grandfather, who taught me how to ride a bike

CONTENTS

SERIES EDITOR'S PREFACE

Global Crises and the Media

We live in a global age. We inhabit a world that has become radically interconnected, interdependent, and communicated in the formations and flows of the media. This same world also spawns proliferating, often interpenetrating, "global crises."

From climate change to the war on terror, financial meltdowns to forced migrations,energy shortages to world poverty, and humanitarian disasters to the denial of human rights, these and other crises represent the dark side of our globalized planet. Their origins and outcomes are not confined behind national borders and they are not best conceived through national prisms of understanding. The impacts of global crises often register across "sovereign" national territories, surrounding regions and beyond, andthey can also become subject to systems of governance and forms of civil society response that are no less encompassing or transnational in scope. In today's interdependent world, global crises cannot be regarded as exceptional or aberrant events only, erupting without rhyme or reason or dislocated from the contemporary world (dis)order. They are endemic to the contemporary global world, deeply enmeshed within it. And so too are they highly dependent on the world's media and communication networks.

The series Global Crises and the Media sets out to examine not only the media's role in the *communication* of global threats and crises but also how they can variously enter into their *constitution*, enacting them on the public stage and helping to shape their future trajectory around the world. More specifically, the volumes in this series seek to: (1) contextualize the study of global crisis reporting and representations in relation to wider debates about the changing flows and formations of world media communication; (2) address how global crises become variously communicated and contested in both so-called "old" and "new" media around the world; (3) consider the possible impacts of global crisis reporting on public awareness, political action, and policy responses; (4) showcase the very latest research findings and discussion from leading authorities in their respective fields of inquiry; and (5) contribute to the development of positions of theory and debate that deliberately move beyond national parochialisms and/or geographically disaggregated research agendas. In these ways the specially commissioned books in the Global Crises and the Media series aim to provide a sophisticated and empirically engaged understanding of the media's changing roles in global crises and thereby contribute to academic and public debate about some of the most significant global threats, conflicts, and contentions in the world today.

The World Health Organization (WHO) identifies emerging and re-emerging epidemic diseases as an on-going threat to global health security. This is not new. It is well known that the Spanish flu in the immediate aftermath of World War I killed over 50 million people, more than those who died on the field of battle. Today we better understand how a new influenza develops from the first few infections to a pandemic. It often begins with a (zoonotic) virus infecting animals before species-leaping and infecting people. It then begins to spread directly throughout the human population and becomes a global pandemic when infections have spread worldwide. In a fast-moving, interconnected and globalized world, the spread of influenza and other mutating, potentially deadly, diseases have become all the more difficult to contain and control. More people now live in urban settings and cities than at any other time in history(over 50%; by 2050 this is expected to grow to 70%). In crowded and squalid urban conditions diseases can easily incubate and spread rapidly. More people are also on the move than at any previous time—for security, for work, or for leisure—within and across national borders and continents. Increasingly many have become internally displaced through war, conflicts, and the environmental impacts of climate change, forcing them to inhabit places that render them vulnerable to increased dangers and risks including outbreaks of disease and epidemics. And the speed and volume of contemporary transport systems, principally aviation, facilitate the movement of vast numbers of people around the planet and in hours not days. The International Air Transport Association (IATA) estimates that in 2013 over 8 million people on average flew every day and over 3 billion across the year. These ever-increasing flights can deposit passengers in the world's major cities before their unsuspecting hosts may even be aware of symptoms of contagious disease. The threats posed by new global pandemics today are all too real.

In 1997 a highly pathogenic strain of avian influenza (HPA1) H5N1 was identified. Severe Acute Respiratory Syndrome (SARS) followed this in 2003. In 2004 HPAI spread from Southeast Asia, reaching Africa and Europe in 2005. The U.S. Centers for Disease Control and Prevention (CDC) estimated the global death toll from the 2009 H1N1 influenza pandemic was more than 284,000. As documented by WHO, 35 million people around the world were living with HIV (human immune deficiency virus) in 2013 and in the same year 1.5 million died of AIDS (acquired immune deficiency). As I write this (August 2014) the deadliest recorded epidemic of Ebola Virus Disease (EVD) is unfolding in West Africa.

It began in Guinea, spreading to Liberia, Sierra Leone, and Nigeria and causing health panics in many major cities (especially those with airports) around the world. In August 2014 WHO recorded a total of 2,615 suspected cases and 1,427 deaths from this terrifying Ebola disease. The Western media, for their part, have reported in depth on the few cases of American and British health workers who contracted the disease and who were flown home on special flights and for emergency treatment in strictly controlled isolation units. Less has been heard about Liberia's West Point in Monrovia and Dolo Town in Margibi, where local populations have been quarantined and placed under full security watch, effectively restricting their movement and confining them inside the outbreak areas.

WHO, the United Nations' supreme world health authority, also formally declared the latest outbreak of EVD as a 'public health emergency of international concern' (PHEIC). This legal designation has only been used twice before (for the 2009 H1N1 'swine flu' pandemic and the 2014 resurgence of polio). The WHO declaration invokes legal measures on disease prevention, surveillance, control, and response, and 194 of the world's nation states are signatories to these measures. How diseases and pandemics become designated, officially responded to, and popularly conceived and understood clearly position them not only as public health concerns but also as potent vehicles for meaning, the conduct of social relations and the discharge of power in and across diverse communities and nations. Myths and meanings in the context of pandemics, it seems, as elsewhere, can prove highly consequential in their symbolic, material, and bodily effects.

It is in this context that *Pandemics and the Media* by Marina Levina provides a timely and entirely welcome addition to the Global Crises and the Media series. As the author states in her introduction, "This book addresses what it means—culturally, politically, and economically—to live in an infected, diseased body, be it a national, a global, or an individual one." Her book offers an original and insightful disquisition on the diverse ways in which contemporary pandemics become culturally constructed and infused with myths and meanings, discourses and narratives, in and through media representations and popular culture and how these enter into hierarchical social relations and processes of 'Othering'. Explorations of the cultural meanings attached to blood, narratives of morality and citizenship in the context of HIV/AIDS, discourses of security in relation to global pandemics, and the cultural metaphors encoded within popular representations of vampires, as well as how new digital media serve to track and visualize pandemics transcending the boundaries of nation-states all feature within this eloquent book. To repeat, how cultural constructs of disease and pandemics enter into the popular imaginary and help to build public responses is not of symbolic consequence only; they become materially encoded and bio-politically embodied in the lives of us all and the life-chances and deaths of too many. I recommend this book to you.

Simon Cottle, Series Editor

ACKNOWLEDGMENTS

This book was written during the time I became a mother to a wonderful and spirited girl. It would not have been possible for me to give birth to a baby and a book at the same time if it were not for an amazing professional and personal support network. It is them that I would like to thank.

Deep gratitude goes to Mary Savigar of Peter Lang and Simon Cottle of the *Global* Crises and *the Media* series for their patience and feedback. My colleagues at the Department of Communication were incredibly supportive throughout this process. I am especially grateful to Leroy Dorsey, our department chair, for understanding the difficulty of balancing life and work for a new parent and for providing a structure of support without which this book would not be finished; Tony de Velasco, for being a wonderful friend and mentor and for helping me navigate the murky waters of pre-tenure existence; Josh Reeves, for support and inspiration, and Nick Simpson, whose companionship kept me sane and smiling. A big thanks goes to my research assistants, Marcus Hassell, Alaenor London, Lindsey Randall, and Jon Paul Bushnell, who provided much-needed help at various parts of this project. Financially, this work was supported in part by grants from College of Communication and Fine Arts New Faculty Grant and The University of Memphis Faculty Research Grant Fund.

This work greatly benefited from the Bright Ideas Visiting Fellowship at the Genomics Forum at the University of Edinburgh, and I am especially grateful to Catherine Lyall and Steve Yearley for making it possible. While there, I was fortunate enough to get invaluable feedback from scholars at The Lancaster University and the University of Exeter, especially Richard Tutton, Maureen McNeil, John Urry, Rebecca Coleman, Adam Fish, Anna Harris, and Michael Morrison. It was only after that visit when I finally knew what the book was about, in no small part thanks to suggestions and enthusiasm of everyone I encountered.

In the larger field of media studies I am fortunate enough to be surrounded by brilliant and supportive friends, advisors, and scholars. I am very thankful to those who kept my spirits up, encouraged me to try again, and demonstrated faith in my ability to write a worthwhile sentence. Especially Radhika Gajjala, Kent Ono, Carol Stabile, Michele White, Rachel Dubrofsky and Craig Robertson for offering words of wisdom and/or a drink when I needed it most. I am profoundly grateful and I hope to be able to pay it forward.

I would not have acclimated to the life in the South if it were not for Laura Daum de Velasco and Sharon Stanley. Their friendship over the last four years has meant the world to me and they inspire me always. Visits and Skype conversations with Ulli Gretzel have been extraordinarily important to my well-being and I want to thank her for being a wonderful friend and the best "second wife" a girl could ask for.

Since this is a book on pandemics, I must thank our family doctor in the Chicago area, Milena Jguenti, a practitioner extraordinaire. Over the past decade she has given me back my health, treated scarlet fever across the Atlantic, and was there for many phone calls and texts on matters large and small. Suffice it to say that, in the case of an outbreak, she would be the first one I call.

I would not have been able to finish this book without support of my family. I am profoundly grateful to my parents Anna Levina and Alex Sher, not just for moving to Memphis and providing extraordinary care to their granddaughter, but for everything they have done for me since we moved to the United States from the former Soviet Union. My mother's strength and charm and my father's kindness and compassion have remained the guiding principles in my life and inspiration for everything that I do. Everything in my life is possible only because of them. My grandmother Fanya, who moved to Memphis at the age of eighty-nine to be near her great-grandaughter, was the first person to help me with math and to show me everything that can be achieved with a little or a lot of perseverance.

In some ways, this acknowledgment is not long enough to properly express the depth of gratitude and love to my husband, Dmitry Ozeryansky. Suffice it to say, that he has taken a bulk of childcare on his shoulders while I was recovering from a c-section and finishing the book. Watching him become an amazing father has been, for me, a great pleasure of the last year. Finally to my daughter Alexandra Eteri Ozeryansky (a.k.a. Sasha), a smart and fearless little girl, whose daily existence is a miracle to me: I hope that Mama will make you proud. She certainly cannot wait to show you the world.

· INTRODUCTION ·

Living in the Pandemic Age

The H1N1 pandemic, also known as the swine flu, started in Mexico in the spring of 2009 and quickly spread to the United States and Canada. While the pandemic was not quite as deadly as some had feared, it did usher in something that *Science* magazine has called the "flu-naming wars" (Enserink, 2009). The fraught negotiations in the scientific, political, cultural, and economic arenas over the proper name for this particular pandemic answered the age-old question, "What's in the name?" Quite a lot, it turns out. The World Health Organization banned the word "swine" from the description of the influenza, renaming it influenza A(H1N1), or as it was shorthanded, H1N1. A spokesman for the Center for Disease Control (CDC) in the United States commented on the name change as a response to sensitive and cultural issues in other parts of the world, as well as issues around the name's impact on commerce in the United States (Grady, 2009). Fiona Fleck, a spokeswoman for the World Health Organization, said that while the virus was originally called swine flu "because the largest component of this new virus was actually swine flu virus.…It doesn't affect pigs, as far as we know. It hasn't been found in pigs. Pigs haven't transmitted it, as far as we know" (Grady, 2009).

In the United States, the name triggered the ire of the pork industry, who feared that it would adversely affect farms and industrial pork production.

Farm groups mounted a campaign to rename the virus "North American influenza" (Martin & Krauss, 2009). The U.S. Department of Agriculture issued a written statement and publically urged the media "to stop calling this 'novel' pandemic virus 'swine flu'" (Falco, 2009). The Department of Agriculture symbolically slapped the news media on the hand for perpetuating the term "swine" flu in reports about the new H1N1 strain of influenza. In a statement posted on the USDA website, USDA secretary Tom Vilsack (2009) pleaded with the media, "Each time the term is used it unfairly hurts America's farmers who are suffering severe economic losses during these challenging economic times. And each time the media uses the phrase 'swine flu' a hog farmer, their workers, and their families suffer. It is simply not fair or correct to associate the 2009 pandemic H1N1 influenza with hogs, an animal that does not play a role in the ongoing transmission of the pandemic strain." And, around the world, the unfortunate name triggered a number of unfortunate responses. Egypt decided to kill all its pigs, about 30,000, even though there were no cases of swine flu in Egypt. The move was quickly criticized by international agencies, even as the press acknowledged that H1N1 was just a convenient excuse for the Egyptian government to get rid of animals that aided *Zabaleen*, a community of people in Cairo and other cities who made their living by collecting and repurposing the city trash (Slackman, 2009). In Israel, meanwhile, Ultra-Orthodox deputy health minister Yaakov Litzman declared that Israel would call the pandemic "Mexico flu" rather than "swine flu," given that pigs are not kosher (Associated Press, 2009). Thailand also decided to call the diseases the "Mexican flu" (Savidge, 2009). The name obviously drew the outrage of the Mexican government, and Mexico's ambassador to Israel, Frederico Salas, registered an official complaint, which prompted a retraction from the Israeli government insisting that it did not plan to change the name of the disease to "Mexican flu" (Pilkington, 2009). These moments of negotiation over the naming, and indeed, the meaning of the pandemic, illustrate two points important to the arguments made in this book: 1) the stories we tell about disease matter; 2) the media are instrumental in constructing and disseminating these stories, and 3) mediated narratives of pandemics are rooted in global flows of policies, commerce, and populations. After all, pandemics are, by definition, global crises.

In her influential book on the HIV/AIDS pandemic, *How to Have a Theory in an Epidemic*, Paula Treichler (1999) calls the meanings, definitions, and attributions produced by HIV/AIDS a semantic epidemic, or an *epidemic of signification*. The term "signification" borrows from the work of Ferdinand de

Saussure, a Swiss linguist who argues that language does not merely describe the world, but rather organizes and gives it meaning. Saussure (1998) argues that the linguistic sign, as comprised by the signifier (a physical representation of the sign) and the signified (a mental representation, or a concept), is arbitrary. In other words, the process of attaching a signified to a signifier is not guided by any inner and discoverable properties of the sign, but rather by the linguistic community, or the culture, in which that articulation takes place. In a simple example, the word "dog," a signifier, and "man's best friend," a signified, only attach together in a specific cultural setting and under particular socioeconomic circumstances. Language, therefore, is a socially constructed entity, subject to myriad political, social, cultural, and economic forces. Barthes (1972) further builds on semiology, or the study of signs, to introduce a second-level semiological system, which he designates "myth." He calls the first system a linguistic system, or the language-object, which myth uses to build its own system, and the second system—myth, or metalanguage—is "a second language in which one speaks about the first" (p. 115). The association between myth and language-object produces the third term of "signification." It is in the process of signification that myth is fully realized through naturalization of that of which it speaks. Barthes writes, "We reach here the very principle of myth: it transforms history into nature.…What causes mythical speech to be uttered is perfectly explicit, but it is immediately frozen into something natural; it is not read as a motive, but as a reason" (p. 129). The language of disease, as mythical speech, naturalizes the historical. Representations of disease are first and foremost historically and culturally based; however, myth converts the historical into the biological and therefore reifies disease as a "natural" phenomenon. In *Madness and Civilization* and *The Birth of the Clinic*, Michel Foucault historicizes and contextualizes the emergence of madness specifically, and of disease in general, as a project of classification and management through various discourses and institutions. He argues that disease has been medicalized through the system of classification, or what he calls "neutralized knowledge." This has changed how we understand disease, infection, and even pain. Foucault (1994) writes, "The figures of pain are not conjured away by means of a body of neutralized knowledge; they have been redistributed in the space in which bodies and eyes meet. What has changed is the silent configuration in which language finds support: the relation of situation and attitude to what is speaking and what is spoken" (p. xi).

Myth, therefore, works at the level of ideology, where certain cultural ideas are reified and presented as natural and obvious. In other words, as

Barthes argues, myth is depoliticized speech. In the cultural and political arenas, a struggle over meaning can therefore be seen as a struggle over signification, a desire to unveil the myth and denaturalize the historical. It is in that arena, according to Treichler, that the contestations of meanings took place during the first decades of the HIV/AIDS pandemic. This was a struggle over the meaning of disease, sexuality, race, and gender. In other words, it was a struggle for signification. Dick Hebdige (1993) describes the struggle for signification as a recognition that social relations and processes are not transparent but are instead shrouded in common sense, which validates and mystifies them. Since all aspects of culture possess a semiotic value, Hebdige argues that "there is an ideological dimension to every signification" (p. 364). Therefore, "[T]he struggle between different discourses, different definitions and meanings within ideology is therefore always, at the same time, a struggle within signification: a struggle for possession of the sign which extends to even the most mundane areas of everyday life" (p. 367). Representation is a signifying practice because it is often a site of contested meanings, ideological struggles, and negotiated difference (Hall et al., 1997). Representations of disease signify various sites of ideological struggles, be it over the image of difference or the portrayal of disease as the loss of control. Sander Gilman (1988), in his study of representations of illness in visual culture, argues that these representations lead to the internalization of cultural predispositions of disease. These predispositions are steeped in cultural constructions of difference, where "the image of the patient is always a playing out of this desire for a demarcation between ourselves and the chaos represented in culture by disease" (p. 4). Similarly, Terry and Urla (1995) argue that disease often represents an *embodied deviance*, or "the term we give to the scientific and popular postulate that the bodies of subjects classified as deviant are essentially marked in some recognizable fashion" (p. 2).

This book is, first and foremost, an engagement with the construction, management, and classification of difference especially in the global context of a pandemic. It is a Foucauldian project insofar as it addresses Michel Foucault's call to look at "how things work at the level of on-going subjugation, at the level of those continuous and uninterrupted processes which subject our bodies, govern our gestures, dictate our behaviors, etc.…We should try to discover how it is that subjects are gradually, progressively, really and materially constituted through a multiplicity of organisms, forces, energies, materials, desires, thoughts, etc. We should try to grasp subjection in its material instance as a constitution of subjects" (Foucault, 1980, p. 97). This book addresses what it means—culturally, politically, and economically—to live in an infected, diseased body, be it a national, a global, or an individual one. It is the preoccupation with the very principle of difference as a material and embodied entity that led me to write this book. I wanted to explore exactly what it means to live, love, and govern in the time of a pandemic in a global environment where flows of commerce, politics, and scientific knowledge are essential to distribution of resources according to previously established principles of difference and otherness. Moreover, if pandemics are an issue of global security, then mediated representations of pandemics constitute subjects in global environments and as a response to global crises. In what Duffield and Waddell (2006) refer to as the biopolitics of global governance, mediated representations are essential in translating and making sense of difference as a category of subjectivity and as a mode of organizing and distributing change.

Using textual analysis, I turn to a broad collection of media texts on pandemics and disease: films, books, television shows, documentaries, public health campaigns, and online pandemic tracking services. These texts, however limited in scope by issues of language and access, are nevertheless representative of a larger mediascape that drafts stories of global instabilities and global health. We can see the struggle over signification as a cultural and mediated determination of which stories are told, which ones acquire the status of authority or truth, and which ones are dismissed outright. These stories are always mediated; in the current mediascape we understand the world predominantly through the eyes of mass media, be it film, television, or the Internet. Priscilla Wald (2008) calls this the *outbreak narrative*:

> That narrative links the idea of disease emergence to worldwide transformations; it interweaves ecological and socioeconomic analysis with a mythic tale of microbial battle over the fate of humanity. The outbreak narrative fuses the transformative force of spaces of global modernity. It also accrues contradictions: the obsolescence and tenacity of borders, the attraction and threat of strangers, and especially the destructive and formative power of contagion. It both acknowledges and obscures the interactions and global formations that challenge national belonging. (p. 33)

In other words, the outbreak narrative encompasses the mythological and ideological properties of language. Wald's conceptualization of the outbreak narrative is exceptionally important to this book. As the reader will notice, I include the horror film genre as an essential part of media pandemic narrative. Throughout my work, I argue that science is in the business of creating narratives that are often elaborate and always fantastic. In the media's retelling of these narratives, the line between science and fiction is blurred. After all, some of the best science in the world reads like science fiction (Levina, 2007). I argue that horror stories of vampires and zombies are essential in our culture's process of determining how diseased and infected bodies get classified and managed in a time of pandemic, as well as defining what it means to survive, and perhaps thrive, as a human or as a monster during a contagion.

I begin this book with a chapter on blood. I argue that a book on pandemics must start with a discussion of blood metaphors because media narratives of pandemics are determined by cultural understanding of infection and contamination, an understanding grounded in social perceptions of blood. In this chapter, I examine evocations of blood as a metaphorical (and literal) site of social and cultural meaning that constructs and manages communities and identities. Chapter two focuses on the HIV/AIDS pandemic in its various cultural contexts. Using theoretical approaches to moral panic, discursive formation, and citizenship, I argue that cultural representations of HIV/AIDS construct narratives of morality and citizenship as categories of inclusion and exclusion in civic life. Chapter three looks at how vampire films have been mapped onto the cultural discourse of HIV/AIDS pandemic. I argue that vampires serve as cultural metaphors for how society classifies and manages diseased and deviant bodies. In chapter four, I explore media representations of global pandemics as social and cultural sites where the problems of governance, security, and risk are presented and resolved. As a global crisis, pandemics demonstrate the anticipatory nature of risk and the immediate biopolitical problem of governance. In chapter five, I go back to monsters, and specifically to cinematic portrayals of zombie pandemics, arguing that zombie outbreaks exemplify the problem of governance during a pandemic and a problem of governing life itself. Finally, I examine digital media pandemic tracking tools and address how digital media construct pandemics as a global problem that transcends the boundaries of nation-states. I argue that, consequently, these technological developments constitute citizens' health in relationship to their online environments and networks in general. Through these various mediated sites, pandemics are represented as sites for change, struggle, and destruction. Ironically enough, they are also sites for determining what, after all, makes us human.

· 1 ·

KEEPING THE BLOOD FLOWING

Disease, Community, and Public Imaginaries

> Blood is liquid life. It is the most intimate liquid and the most powerful medicine all of us can give and hope to receive. The idea of blood reaches deep into our consciousness. If you look at the history of blood, it is really the history of self-discovery of the human race. In the modern age to give blood is a powerful act of human charity, a universal expression of self-sacrifice in peace or war or in the face of disaster. Blood permeates all aspects of life, because blood is life. For better or worse if you control blood, you control life itself.

So begins PBS documentary *Red Gold: The Epic Story of Blood.* A four-hour documentary first aired in November 2002, it unfolds partly as a continuous Red Cross advertisement for blood donation, and partly as a story of communities created and destroyed by blood practices. Each hour-long section (*Magic to Medicine*, *Blood and War*, *Tainted Blood*, *New Blood*) reveals a multitude of cross-sections between blood research, social practices, scientific and historical change, and popular imagination. Along the way, it evokes the literal and figurative mysteries, the rituals, and the promises and dangers of blood. The documentary is based on the book by Douglas Starr titled *Blood: An epic history of medicine and commerce* (2002), and the author is on hand to structure much of the narrative. The documentary's argument is that blood science, while frequently beneficial, is always potentially dangerous. It repeatedly argues that blood is either liquid life or a contaminated harbinger of death. This chapter uses the *Red Gold* documentary to examine how the media uses blood as a category to demarcate contaminated bodies and to construct public health campaigns that manage the boundaries of communities and nation-states. A book on pandemics must start with a discussion of blood metaphors because media narratives of pandemics are determined by cultural understanding of infection and contamination. And that understanding is grounded in social perceptions of blood.

In this book I examine *how* bodies (and by extension communities and identities organized around these bodies) are *drawn together* and managed by popular and scientific discourses. Therefore, what is at stake in discussion of the metaphors of blood science is the construction and management of the body. I look at what metaphors *do* and what they do for those who employ, exploit, and deploy them. In this chapter, I examine evocations of blood as a metaphorical (and literal) site of social and cultural meaning that constructs and manages communities and identities. I argue that blood is both a boundary liquid that functions to demarcate difference and a powerful instrument for building community and identity. That duality frames how blood boundaries are created, used, and maintained. Cultural narratives of blood manage difference through scientific and cultural exclusion and/or incorporation. In the process, certain struggles, sufferings, and deaths are assigned more gravitas than others. What emerges is a homogeneous account of a community that employs difference as a point of reference to itself: *We do not have bad, tainted, evil blood, and therefore we are good, innocent or righteous*. Moreover, I argue that the metaphors of blood as life position blood as a totalizing entity that essentializes body and identity. It is only in this context that metaphors such as "bad blood" can make sense. It implies that identity is inextricably tied to blood. As such identity is perceived as a static force, for our blood penetrates every part of our body and cannot be easily replaced. Through the use of metaphors, blood transcends its particular physiological function in the human body and becomes a signifier for matters of life and death. But despite such large themes, blood and its narratives are vulnerable to history and politics. Blood is not life. It is a liquid inside bodies that has been used, metaphorically or literally, but always socially, to create communities, manage differences, further scientific careers, and justify various politics of exclusion. And as such, blood narratives are a contested battleground of meaning. In his cultural history of hematology, Keith Wailoo (1997) writes:

> When the 19th century hematologist took the blood as his focus, he chose a rich symbol of individual identity, social health, and group relations.…Even with the increasing specialization of medicine, blood study continued to have metaphorical appeal, offering the practitioner a role as a "secret agent"—producer of both specific and generalized knowledge.…Whether because of habit or because "power speaks *through* blood"(Foucault, 1978/1990), this fluid has continued to be mysterious and potent, containing for doctor and patient alike a wealth of vital yet hidden information about disease, the body, and society.…The history of hematology is also a history of creating of the identity—patient, doctor, disease identity. To study this relationship—the construction and management of disease identities and medical identities—is not simply to reject, a priori, these constructions. It is, rather, to see these constructions as dynamic entities, shaping medical practice and social behavior, evolving with the cultural relations of bio-medicine, and existing alongside (and often in conflict with) experiential, social, political, or spiritual constructions of self and disease (pp. 6, 13).

Much scholarship has been dedicated to studying the role of blood in constructing racial (Tapper, 1999; Wailoo, 2001; Weston, 2001, etc.), national (Linke, 1999; Marvin & Ingle, 1999; White, 1993, etc.), and public health crises (Bayer, 1999; Feldman, 1999; Fontaine, 2002; Wailoo, 1997, etc.). Dorothy Nelkin, in her investigation of cultural perspectives on blood, identifies four repeated and related themes around which blood metaphors cluster: blood as the essence of personhood, blood exchange practices as a symbol of community solidarity, blood as a source of danger and risk, and finally, "the concept of pure blood contains associations that extend well beyond the properties of a biological substance to include references to social relationships and moral as well as physical contamination" (Nelkin, 1999, p. 275). In this chapter I loosely build upon Dorothy Nelkin's metaphorical categories to systematically analyze how blood is constructed as a category to demarcate contaminated bodies and construct media campaigns that manage boundaries of communities and nation-states.

Blood and Life Itself

> Blood in our veins remains a powerful symbol of identity and vitality. The gift of life itself. Many of its mysteries have been solved, but one central challenge remains: how to provide ourselves with enough of our lifeblood, our red gold.…Blood still holds in the collective psyche, as it has throughout history. Lifeblood, one's essence. And so the giving of that has been seen as something precious. And it continues to be so.

So ends the documentary. Its first section—*Magic to Medicine*—tells the story of Jean-Baptiste Denis, a physician to Louis XIV, who believed that the essential characteristics of a person or an animal were carried in their blood, and that one could therefore cure madness through transfusion with a calm animal's blood. In 1667, he transfused the blood of a calf into a manic patient. The patient went into a state of shock and became extremely ill. For at least a period of time after the experiment, however—probably as a result of a nearly fatal experience—he was no longer manic. Detractors, fueled by scientific jealousy, argued that to interfere with the sacred blood of life was an abomination, but Denis declared the experiment a success (Starr, 1998). Even so, the view that blood transfusion could potentially change a person's essence was common, and informed much of the earlier blood experiments.

Blood was considered to be the seat of the soul, and it was thought that the body was rejuvenated through various forms of consumption of young and innocent blood. For example, the sixteenth-century surgeon Jean Tagault observed that by good blood the flesh was renewed, the good blood being "vicious neither in quality nor in quantity" (Camporesi, 1995, p. 19). According to Camporesi, around the same time, "physicians, apothecaries, charlatans, and great intellectuals [of the day] all agreed: the blood of a fresh, delicate man, one well-tempered in his humors, someone young, soft, and blooming with red, 'bloody' fat—a fleshy man, of a 'jovial' temperament and 'cordial' character, preferably having red hair [association with the color of blood]—enjoyed the indisputable primacy when it came to the slowing of the aging process" (p. 17). The mythology is plentiful: the ancient Egyptians bathed in blood to regain youth; witches in the Middle Ages were thought to drink blood of the young to keep their power, and vampires were thought to drink blood in order to keep themselves alive. Nicolae Ceausescu, the infamous hypochondriac Romanian dictator, was rumored to keep little boys in his castle in order to draw blood from them periodically for his own rejuvenation (Nelkin, 1999). Despite the detractors of such practices, the obsession with the blood of the young illustrates the belief that by consuming someone's blood, one would also consume the essence of that person. This belief structured early experiments in transfusion. Oxford's "Experimental Philosophers Club," described in the documentary, first injected alcohol into a dog's blood and then transfused its blood into another dog to see if the alcohol-tinted blood would affect another animal. Although it is not explicitly stated in the documentary, the purpose was to experiment with essence—of the animal, and then of the human. In the documentary, historian Kim Pelis describes the debate over "what would happen if we transfuse between humans, between animals and humans. "What would happen," Samuel Pepys asked, "if we would transfuse the blood of a Quaker in the Archbishop?" The metaphor of blood as a self's essence informed much of the modern political, legal, scientific, and social development. And, as a politically significant metaphor, blood was used to construct and classify numerous social categories of identity.

Media representations of blood, as seen here, use metaphors of blood as essence of life to tell a story of a self which is defined through both blood and its associated practices. Each metaphor—a mapping of one conceptual domain onto another—is an important theoretical guidepost as well (Bright, 1992). Since any given concept can be described in many ways, a metaphor gives defining qualities to that concept. By encouraging focus on one aspect of a concept, a metaphor directs attention away from other aspects, especially those inconsistent with that metaphor (Lakoff & Johnson, 2003). It is the metaphor, rather than the concept, that shapes perceptions and actions. As Lakoff and Johnson (2003) put it, "[M]etaphors may create realities for us, especially social realities. A metaphor may thus be a guide for future action. Such actions will, of course, fit the metaphor. This will, in turn, reinforce the power of the metaphor to make experience coherent. In this sense metaphors can be self-fulfilling prophecies" (p. 156). For example, defining blood as life itself invites different perceptions and activities than does the metaphor of blood as the harbinger of death. The former invites donation, the latter fear over sharing, bleeding, and contact. Each of these activities then reinforces the associated metaphor. The metaphor of blood as life's essence is also problematic in other ways. It seems to mean everything when, in fact, it means nothing. Life, as a concept, only acquires meaning within a particular social, historical, and cultural context. When "life" is given no specific historical meaning, then "life"—much like "God"—becomes a transcendental signified (Derrida, 1978; 1997). Positioned outside a particular historical context, it nevertheless determines the meaning of any narrative to which it is related. Therefore blood as life justifies social and political actions. If blood is the essence of life itself then the desire to protect it can be used to justify a variety of questionable objectives. In the rest of the chapter, I illustrate how a representation of blood as life was used by different public health campaigns to justify community actions, persecutions, and even death.

Pure Blood

Over the footage of blond youths, taken from Nazi propaganda films of the 1930s, *Red Gold* describes the Nazi belief that the pure-blooded Aryan super race was rooted in the very soil of the German fatherland. The movement's slogan, "Blood and Soil," was thus literal as well as symbolic. Indeed, a group of Nazi doctors who called themselves the German Blood Group Society set out to establish a scientific link between blood and soil. The research of the Polish serologist Ludwig Hirszfeld during the World War I era suggested the inhabitants of certain geographical regions frequently share some blood groups but not others. While Hirszfeld avoided connecting the frequency of blood groups to generalizations about race, and condemned the Nazis' use of his findings, the Society pursued its own thesis (Starr, 1998). Having produced a map showing a concentration of blood group A in Germany and blood group B in Eastern Europe, they argued that blood group A was in danger of being polluted by the inferior blood group B. In the documentary, Dr. Pauline Mazumdar, a historian at the University of Toronto, explains: "The idea was that they could associate blood group A with Aryan and that the great Aryan race was at home on German soil. Blood group B was an ideologically loaded group that encapsulated Jews, Gypsies, Slavs, and other undesirables. Many people interested in blood groups were bacteriologists, so the idea of infection spreading across the countryside from the East was something that bacteriologists were familiar with." Even before the advent of the Nazi regime, unspecified German studies had concluded that blood-type A individuals were more athletic and that blood-type B individuals spent more time on the toilet (Starr, 1998). Nazi Germany was not the only place where blood groups were considered to possess certain personality characteristics. For example, in Japan, many people believe that blood type determines personal character, and is a template of identity. Blood-type analyses are used, both playfully and seriously, to predict personality and behavior. Magazine profiles of political candidates include information about their blood types, dating services use blood analysis to make matches, and mismatched blood types have been grounds for divorce. There are condoms that indicate blood types. Even in anime, blood types of characters are often listed.

Kevles (2001) argued that the nature of blood-group research lent itself to the research on protection and management of population. He writes,

> Blood groups provided precisely the kind of unambiguous trait that human geneticists like to find.…A different use of blood-group data has been suggested during

> the First World War when the Polish serologist Ludwig Hirszfeld had sampled sixteen different people in that polyglot area [Macedonia] and demonstrated that the distribution of the four blood groups then known varied from one ethnic population to another. By the 40s, increasing refinement in the identification of blood groups... permitted drawing detailed serological profiles of distinct populations and determining their degree of intermixture. Blood-group genetics thus joined ethnography, anthropology, and demography as a valuable tool in the study of human history, particularly migrations and mixings, and ultimately of human evolution. (p. 197)

Eugenics, in this sense, can be seen as a classification project that used blood and descent as interlaced categories to define individual and social bodies and identities. In fact, the word "eugenics" was coined in 1883 by Francis Galton and comes from a Greek root meaning "good in birth" or "noble in heredity." Kevles (2001) writes, "[Galton] intended it to denote the 'science' of improving human stock by giving the more suitable races of strains of blood a better chance of prevailing speedily over the less suitable" (p. xiii). Before a decision can be made about what to do with the "infected," they must first be defined, identified, and organized. For eugenics, blood was a useful organizational tool because it embodied "the essence" of a person (racial, ethnic, or otherwise) and therefore provided a totalizing account of that person's identity based on group membership. Eugenics in this light can be seen as a quintessential modern narrative that foregrounds the beliefs in the essential nature of "man," progress, and nationhood. Here, blood serves as a useful tool for control of the nation-state's literal and metaphorical boundaries. As Jeffrey Weeks (1995) argues, the study of eugenics was based on assumptions that "inferior" races would hinder the economic and imperial expansion of Western nations. In fact, the "Blood and Soil" campaign wanted to ensure the cleanliness of German boundaries against foreign infections of bodies and characters.

Uli Linke (1999) cites Adolf Hitler's assertion that blood is unchangeable and eternal: "[C]lasses vanish, classes alter themselves, the destinies of men undergo changes, but something always remains: the nation as such, as the substance of flesh and blood. To us [National Socialists] blood not only means something corporeal, but it is in a racial sense, the soul, which has as its external field of expression the body." The slogan "Blood and Soil" was a nationalist project that linked German identity with the soil and peasant identity. Peasants, or *volk*, working on the land, were seen as authentically German and an essential blood source for the nation (Linke, 1999). At the root of the "Blood and Soil" project was an attempt to counteract the influence of the cities, with their many opportunities for intermarriage and sexual contact across races. To control such activities, many educational programs were put in place to instruct people in matters of heredity, marriage, and sex. Linke (1999) mentions a number of proverbs that were published in the Nazi folklore journal *Volk und Rasse* in 1936 under the title "Living Racial Hygiene in the German Proverb":

> Only those who are alike should exchange their hands in marriage.
> Race sticks to race
> To marry into the blood (close relative) is seldom good [blood identity should not encompass incest]
> The closer to the blood, the worse the offspring [ibid.]
> It is in the blood, if it was in the clothes, one could brush it out.
> Three things make the best couples: same blood, same passion, and same age.
> First healthy blood, then a large estate and a pretty hat. (qtd. in Linke, 1999, p. 206)

Bodies were disciplined—through marriage and the regulations of sexual activities, educational programs, racial segregation, and even death—according to the doctrine of blood as a source of an individual's essence. Descent was defined in terms of blood; the definitional notion of race was based on blood, not on a person's color or religious beliefs (Scales-Trent, 2001). Jewishness was not defined according to religious practices, but according to the "one drop of blood" rule. In March 1936 *Der Sturmer* wrote, "Whoever has Jewish blood in his veins will sooner or later reveal the Jewish part of his character" (Miller, 1995). But blood as a classification tool, used to patrol boundaries of bodies and nations, was not solely reserved for Nazi policies. It also informed American racial policies of the time.

The documentary briefly discusses the exclusion of African Americans from blood donation during World War II. The most significant comment on the topic in the documentary is made by Keith Wailoo, a historian at Rutgers University: "African Americans as a group were treated or regarded in much of the same way as Typhoid Mary…as a potential carrier of all sort of maladies that could be transmitted through miscegenation, through touching, or simply by walking down the street." This reflected the fears of "catching black" that permeated American culture at the time, fears steeped in the belief in the essentialist properties of blood. For example, Eva Saks (1989) writes that "race categories in American have long been based on ideas about 'blood quanta'… African Americans were identified by the one drop of blood rule,' which defined a person with even a drop of 'black blood' as black.…[In the American South] miscegenation laws used the metaphor of 'black blood' to separate the legal concept of race from skin color. The skin could lie, allowing a person to pass, but the blood represented 'serological truth'; it defined and identified race" (Saks, 1989, pp. 29–41). Thus, the body was racialized using blood as the predominant classification tool. The cultural representation of sickle cell anemia, which occurs predominantly in African American populations, illustrates the use of race to manage, discipline, and treat the body. As Melbourne Tapper (1999) argues, "[S]ickling today is viewed as a black-related disease not simply because the majority of people suffering from the disease are blacks, but because various medical sciences in tandem with anthropology have represented it as a disease of 'black people' since the turn of the twentieth century" (p. 3). Until the 1940s, sickle cell anemia was viewed as a disease of "Negro blood" that can be passed on to the white population through interracial relationships (Wailoo, 1997). As Wailoo points out, this was not a simple matter of "bad" or "prejudiced" science. The existence of racially identifiable blood was a real material experience for both physicians and patients. He writes, "for many physicians in the early 20th century, 'Negro blood' was a term with clear technological origins and with biological, social, and public health meanings. These physicians based their view on what was at that time hematological evidence and scientific understanding of…the disorder" (p. 137). Regardless of a patient's symptoms or claims of racial whiteness, sickle cells, and therefore, "Negro blood", were there, in the body, waiting to be found. Since mere visual evidence could not be trusted to identify "true" racial identities, bodies were once again classified according to their genealogies or descent. But, as Tapper (1999) points out, even when black ancestry could be ruled out for three or five generations, doctors were still unable to accept their subjects' claim to be "racially pure whites."

One issue at stake in these negotiations and narratives is kinship. Through the use of blood as a classification category, alliances are drawn, boundaries are established, and brotherhoods are declared. Franklin and McKinnon (2001) write, "[A]s a classificatory technology, kinship can be mobilized to signify not only specific kinds of connection and inclusion but also specific kinds of disconnection and exclusion" (p. 15). They argue that kinship presents historically contingent knowledge as primordial, natural facts. Thus the language of descent in Nazi Germany (as well as in the United States) transformed sociological categories of race into biological "truths" (Scales-Trent, 2001). In short, kinship authorizes a search for origins that offers up a "natural" reality, which then must be guarded against intrusions. For example, Tapper (1999) details the search for the origin of sickle cell anemia that took doctors Thomas B. Cooley and Pearl Lee to Africa in the mid-1920s. In the process, Tapper argues, Africa was constituted as a kind of primordial reality. He writes, "[T]he African body was deemed likely to hold the key to the true 'racial' and biological nature of its derivate, the "Negro" body.... Sickling among 'Negroes' in the United States could not be fully understood, it was implied, until an account of sickling among Africans had been made" (p. 334). Cooley and Lee's quest established a link between tribe and blood and the use of blood as a valid marker of supposed tribal identity. Tapper continues, "To the external criteria of similarity and difference [that defined the tribe as an identifiable group of people] had been added a criterion from the archives of the body—the blood picture (sickling status) of individual tribespeople. The tribe, in short, had been naturalized" (p. 347). Kinship also shapes social practices of blood sharing and community building. Therefore the claim "it's in the blood" is extended from individual to social bodies. This metaphor organizes nations, citizenships, and, as I have argued, racial and ethnic affiliations. Public health narratives of blood donation practices are an effort to create a seamless narrative of community participation and sacrifice. In the next section, I turn my attention to blood as a site for building community, society, and nationhood. I focus on public health campaigns promoting blood donation during World War II as an example of how social blood practices produced and managed the individual and social body.

Blood and Community

One of the ways in which blood was used to build communities was the Red Cross blood drive. Conducted during times of crisis, such as World War II, the Red Cross used narratives of patriotism, nationalism, and unity to solicit donations. However, the drive also served as a powerful mechanism of exclusion. It divided blood, and therefore blood donors, into those included in the narratives of nationhood and those excluded. *Red Gold* alludes to the treatment of African Americans blood donation during World War II:

> Not everyone in America could join in the flow of blood and patriotism. Some were excluded, even from the self-sacrifice that the nation asked....For years it was assumed that racial identity was contained literally in the blood although there was no scientific basis for such a notion....In the war against racist Nazi enemy, America was forced to confront its own policy of racial discrimination between African Americans and whites. Segregation was common in the 1940s America. Should blood be segregated too?

Clashes over blood donation policies are by no means unique to the American context. In 1996, it was disclosed that Israel's blood banks had a secret policy of destroying blood donated by Ethiopian-Israelis supposedly due to a high level of HIV infection in that population. No evidence of the infection rate was provided and protesters carried signs with slogans like "My blood is as red as yours" (Bartholet, 1996; Kaplan, 1998). In other words, blood donation continues to be a contested ground on which national, cultural, social, and individual identities are negotiated. It can be argued that exclusion from blood donation is metaphorically equivalent to exclusion from the community (Nelkin, 1999). The documentary briefly laments the exclusion, and eventual segregation, of African Americans from blood donation during World War II. But blood donation did not and does not function only as a process of inclusion or exclusion, but also as a process of managing and disciplining individual bodies to be functioning parts of the social. In the management process the social body is defined and organized by both practices and discourses. In this sense the social body is not a product of consensus but rather of material power operating on individual bodies (Foucault, 1980).

For example, Amy Fairchild's book *Science at the Borders* (2003) illustrates how discourses of health and disease served to organize the influx of immigrants into the United States at the turn of the twentieth century. She argues that the overarching purpose of the physical exams administered to the incoming immigrants was not to exclude, but to control how and to what degree immigrants would be incorporated into the social body. For example, in 1905 "poor physique" was the third most common reason for an undesired medical certification. When the Immigration Services asked Dr. J.W. Schereschewsky, stationed in Baltimore, to provide a more precise definition of this category, he "produced for the agency a definition that rested on a broad notion of citizenship, incorporating not only fears about industrial fitness, and thus class fitness, but also and more directly fears about racial unsuitability for participation in democracy.…Poor physique" meant that "the alien concerned is afflicted with a body not only ill adapted to the work necessary to earn his bread, but also poorly able to withstand the onslaught of disease." He "is undersized, poorly developed, with feeble heart action, arteries below the standard size; that he is physically degenerate, and as such not only unlikely to become a desirable citizen, but also very likely to transmit his undesirable qualities to his offspring should he, unfortunately for the country in which he is domiciled, have any" (p. 166). In 1910 the commissioner general of immigration used that definition to argue that the country should demand a high level of physical fitness from its immigrants: "Any measure that will tend...to raise the standard of physical excellence ought to meet with the approval of all citizens who are anxious to preserve and improve the American race....This is not only a question of the present; it is more distinctly a matter of grave concern for the future. The strength of a nation is the combined strength of its individual members. Can we expect, if we continue to inject into the veins of our nation the blood of ill-formed, undersized persons, as are so many of the immigrants now coming, that the American of to-morrow will be the sturdy man he is to-day?" (Fairchild, 2003, p. 168).

Much like the example above, practices of blood donation can be read as a part of the process of creating a model, unified, and disciplined social body. Blood donation posters illustrate this point. In these posters, donors are portrayed as happy and willing, their arms are extended forward, their bodies conform to a life-affirming experience. These posters, featuring people of different races and ethnicities, reinforce the message that everyone is welcome to donate blood. However, donor bodies also conform to the standards of civilized social bodies—they are usually professional, clean-cut, and well dressed. They are not just model donors, but also model citizens. Slogans, such as "Become one of the special people," imply an exclusive, yet readily accessible, community of blood donors. Posters portraying those receiving donated blood mirror those of the donors. Recipients are portrayed with their arms extended, much like donors. There are usually intimate details that introduce a personal relationship and a glimpse into that person's life. The implicit message seems to be, "Now that you know him, give him blood." Recipients are usually "average" people—if they need blood donation, it is implied, then you could, too. A family member, usually a woman, also often sits by them. These public health promotions evoke WWII Red Cross posters that urged civilians to help soldiers through various home-front activities, including blood donation. These posters picture a clean-cut, all-American soldier with a Red Cross female worker at his side. The woman is the home front; she represents a nurturing community. The slogan says, "Now, more than ever—your Red Cross is by his side." The soldier is a wounded hero and a parallel is drawn between wounded heroes and blood donors. Their poses suggest openness and an invitation to the community to become part of their lives.

For its part, *Red Gold* tells a story of blood donation as a principal tool for nation building. Drawing on the history of blood donation during WWII and the advertising of the Red Cross blood donation program, the documentary directly connects an individual act of blood donation to the health and security of the nation. This narrative transcends blood donation as a medical act and instead, portrays the act as a process of incorporating difference into a unified social body. Even those excluded from blood donation did not question the connection between blood donation and nation building. The documentary's coverage of the blood donation in World War II constructs narratives of a "model" and "civilized" donor body that actively, and voluntarily, participates in a unifying ritual of blood donation. In the process, the ideas and ideals of citizenship and nationhood are played out on the individuals' bodies. *Red Gold* argues that blood donations served an instrumental role in community-building during World War II. The posters encouraging WWII home-front effort captioned drawings of soldiers with slogans like "While someone gives his life—what are you giving?" and "Your blood can save him." A poster of the actor Clark Gable in the military uniform carries the slogan "Capt. Clark Gable's message: The RED CROSS is there when *your* soldier needs *you*." In the documentary, Roy Popkins, former Red Cross PR manager, says, "it's [blood donation] something very personal you could do. It was almost like reaching out and giving that soldier a big hug." Public campaigns affirmed the bond between soldiers in the field and blood donors on the home front with slogans such as "Keep your Red Cross at his side" and "A pint of your blood may save a soldier's life." Blood was portrayed as a safety net for the "fallen soldier" and blood donation was a moral equivalent to spilling blood on the battlefield.

Blood united countries as well. In *Red Gold*, over images of the Blitzkrieg, a voiceover says, "From across the Atlantic, Americans watched Britain's plight with dismay and wanted to help. America was not yet in the war, but there was a powerful and symbolic gift that it could make....Britain would always need more blood." This description brushed over America's continuing neutrality as the lives of millions in Europe were under attack and ascribed to blood donation the same symbolic impact as a full military participation in the war. Blood donation became a form of community unification, national war effort, and patriotism, which was by no means unique to the United States. As the documentary points out, even prior to WWII, in Britain blood donations were seen as a source of national pride. Percy Lane Oliver, a doctor in London, invented the world's first voluntary blood donor panels, or "donors-on-the-hoof," a network of donors who were on call twenty-four hours a day. The documentary includes interviews with two men who were donors-on-the-hoof for fifty years. They are shown traveling around town and revisiting old places of glory. One of the men, Jeffrey, says, "I gave some forty-odd blood donations and I qualified for a triple bypass eight years ago and as a part of that procedure I got six pints back. A very good bargain I thought." As WWII put unprecedented demands on blood collection, mobilization efforts relied heavily on a symbolic equivalence of blood, community, and patriotism. Prior historical struggles were also evoked. The donor certificate in Britain included a famous line from Shakespeare's *Henry V*: "For he today that sheds his blood with me / Shall be my brother."

Symbolic associations between blood and community partially explain *Red Gold*'s treatment of the Soviet Union's research into the use of cadaver blood. The documentary represents this practice as something that could only exist outside of civilized Western reason. The story begins with a dramatization of two doctors drinking tea and saluting a portrait of Stalin on the wall. This mood-establishing image is accompanied by generic Russian folk music. The voiceover states, "A revolutionary, but extremely macabre answer to the problem of giving blood on the hoof was developed at the Main Emergency Hospital in Moscow in the 1930s. In the brave new world of the Soviet Union, pride in the latest medical innovation glowed brightly like a Communist dream....It was an idea that could have been spawned in the morbid imagination of a Russian novelist." Scientist Sergey Yudin's very successful experiments with transfusing fresh cadaver's blood are represented by the documentary as outside of Western sensibility and as indicative of morbid fascination with death. These representations of blood-collection practices distinguish the civilized from the barbaric. For example, in the documentary, Dr. Percy Lane Oliver, who ran wartime donor panels in Britain, is quoted as saying that the British temperament has a strong aversion to making use of the corpse. Direct associations are drawn between Soviet medicine and Aldous Huxley's *Brave New World*, again naturalizing Western reaction to this practice without questioning how many lives it could have saved. British and American responses to these experiments—in one case, a British doctor said that "We prefer to keep our blood in people"—further indicate that the use of cadaver blood transgressed the limits of what was considered appropriate in a crisis. The documentary website explains, "It is doubtful that transfusions with blood secured from cadavers could ever have been employed in any country in the world except Russia, for the idea, in spite of its logic, is revolting" (Blood Type, n.d.). In short, while the Soviet Union's method of blood collection saved lives, it did not aim to build communities and nations and, therefore, was deemed inadequate and even barbaric.

René Girard (1979), in his famous study of violence and the sacred, argues that the symbolic connection between blood, ritual, and sacrifice can serve to cleanse communities of the perpetual cycle of violence. He writes:

> How can one cleanse the infected members of all trace of pollution? Does there exist some miraculous substance potent enough not only to resist infection but also to purify, if need be, the contaminated blood? Only blood itself, blood whose purity has been guaranteed by the performance of appropriate rites—the blood, in short, of sacrificial victims—can accomplish this feat (p. 36).

Indeed, Marvin and Ingle (1999) argue that war can be considered both a cycle of violence and a purification ritual. And although soldiers are the primary sacrificial victims of that ritual, the entire community needs to participate in order for the ritual to be effective. Therefore, blood donation can be looked at as a metaphorical blood-spilling that makes civilians into at least partial sacrificial victims and unites the community through this act of purification. For example, during WWII, blood donors were awarded "emblems," a stand-in for medals: bronze for the first donation, silver for the third donation, and a gold-colored "emblem" for the members of the "Gallon Club" (Chinn, 2000). Chinn also shows that wartime blood donation effort emphasized the "averageness" of donors. These stories of "real" Americans participating in the war effort made war heroes of civilians. This translated into what Chinn calls "the mutuality of American identity," the establishment of a relationship between donor and recipient based on shared identity. The American Red Cross's Dedication Label Plan furthered this symbolic relationship between donors and soldiers by enabling donors to label blood with their own name. The Red Cross stated in its documents that "labels on the plasma must necessarily be symbolic, since the individual's blood loses its identity in the laboratory processing" (Chinn, 2000, p. 122). Labeling visually connects blood to a donor body and therefore suggests an imaginary, yet powerful, kinship or alliance between donor and recipient.

The conflation of blood and nationhood in WWII occurred in a multitude of ways. Lieutenant General John L. Dewitt, who was largely responsible for the deportation of Japanese Americans from the Pacific coast, argued that the impossibility of determining Japanese loyalty necessitated evacuation. His 1943 report argued that "the Japanese race is an enemy race and while many second- and third-generation Japanese born of the United States soil, possessed of United States citizenship, have become 'Americanized,' the racial strains are undiluted" (Chinn, 2000, p. 134). This was a veiled reference to the Japanese rule of *jus sanguinis* (the right of blood), which held that children of Japanese parents were Japanese nationals, no matter where they were born because—by this law—Japan had claim on their blood (Chinn, 2000). This illustrates an interesting juxtaposition between citizenship (as a self-chosen identification) and nationality (as an "authentic" identity written in a person's blood).

The issues raised in these letters are echoed in the official histories as well. According to the official report issued by the Office of the Surgeon General in 1964 and titled *Blood Program in World War II*, the Red Cross initial policy for blood donation during WWII specified, "[D]onations should be accepted from both males and females and from members of all races." The report, based on data from Dr. G. Canby Robinson's final report of the Red Cross Blood Donor Service in July 1946, does not mention refusal or segregation of donor blood. *The Compact History of the American Red Cross*, however, provides another account of WWII practices:

> By public demand, as registered with the military, blood was labeled as to race of the donor so that, to put it nicely, a recipient might receive blood from a member of his own race....Chairman Davis...issue[d] public statements to the effect that the Red Cross was following its mandate from the Army and Navy, that it was not the responsibility of the Red Cross "to try to settle racial controversies." In retrospect it appears that the Red Cross could have taken no other course. (Hurd, 1959, p. 227)

Foster Rhea Dulles in *The American Red Cross: A History*, published in 1950, notes that the ARC's original policy toward WWII blood donation was to exclude black donors altogether. After much protest by the African American groups, the policy was amended to segregation. The ARC stated, "In deference to the wishes of those for whom the plasma is being provided, the blood will be processed separately so that those receiving transfusions may be given plasma from the blood of their own race" (p. 420). Dulles writes, "Although medical authorities were agreed that there was no difference whatsoever between Negro and white blood, both Red Cross and Government officials were convinced that regardless of scientific opinion, there would be so much opposition to mixing the blood of white and colored persons that such a procedure would deprive the blood donor program of the universal support essential for it success....In upholding Red Cross policy, Chairman Davis... raised the further question of whether 'under a Democracy...the wishes or prejudices of those who are to receive the blood [white troops] should prevail or the wishes of a relatively small percentage of those who wish to give their blood [black donors]'" (p. 420). Dulles cites former Red Cross chairperson

Livingston Farran, who, twenty years earlier and under different circumstances, had said, "The Red Cross has no 'social theories,' it has only social practices" (p. 421). Dulles continues, "The criticism of this discriminatory feature of its blood donor program was basically a criticism of the workings of American democracy" (p. 421). Blood donation as a social practice goes to the core of how the social will be defined as a category and how individual bodies will be interpellated and managed by the social.

In its coverage of the events following the attacks of 9/11, *Red Gold* evokes again the WWII spirit of blood donation, sacrifice, and community renewal. This exposition works as a Red Cross public service announcement, but it also communicates the symbolic, if not practical, importance of blood donation. It points out that September 11th prompted more blood donations in the United States, and around the world, than any other crisis. While the high casualty rate meant that there was no practical need for blood donation, the documentary reaffirmed the symbolic importance of the practice through the story of Paul Brown, a "model" donor who gives blood on monthly basis. He is shown on the Brooklyn Bridge looking onto the site where the two towers used to stand. His own voiceover narrates, "Blood still holds in the collective psyche, as it has throughout history. Lifeblood; one's essence. And so the giving of that has been seen as something precious. And it continues to be so" (2002). An interesting point: Paul Brown is an African American. The documentary obviously wanted to show the inclusion of all races in our enlightened age. He is represented as a "model" donor, someone who reaffirms community bonds through the practice of blood donation. His body fully participates in the American society and his identity is incorporated into the general category of "American." In the process, the documentary makes his race a nonissue and therefore erases the historical, cultural, and social forces that went into shaping such blood practices.

Moreover, blood donation is reaffirmed, not for its practical benefits, but for the metaphorical and symbolic community rituals that it evokes. Douglas Starr, in an article published after the airing of *Red Gold*, voices a sharp critique of Red Cross's collection of blood in the wake of 9/11. He charges that large amounts of blood were wasted, money was overspent, and general confidence in the Red Cross as an organization was put at risk:

> The events confirmed something that people in the blood business had long known but never managed to communicate to the public: Mass appeals for blood after a crisis may soothe our sense of wounded nationhood and answer a need for community action; but as a public health response, the practice is useless or worse. (Starr, 2002, p. 13)

Blood donation, however, is not only a life-reaffirming practice. As it was discussed earlier, it can also become a "harbinger of death." In the next section, I examine blood donation and blood products became associated with the dangerous body of the Other.

Blood and Danger

Red Gold first represents the dangers of blood through the monstrous imaginary. Kim Pelis, a medical historian, analyzes a montage of a red alcove filled with fire, in front of which a large body—supposedly that of Frankenstein's monster—is rising from the stretcher: "Blood and electricity at that time are both thought to be vital materials. Something that preserves life in the material of blood and electricity…something that can reverse death itself" (2002). James Blundell—a nineteenth-century pioneer in blood-transfusion research—wrote about one of his experiments that a woman was "reanimated as by electric blood." Placing blood transfusion into the realm of Frankenstein-like reanimations, the documentary reaffirms metaphors of blood as a mysterious, unknown, and possibly dangerous liquid.

The documentary draws a parallel between Blundell's experiments and vampire metaphors: "A year after Blundell performed his first transfusion, the first vampire novel was published. The blood-sucking demon was a sinister counterpart to the life-saving transfusers of blood. The culture seems to [be] speaking up about humanity interfering with our own life blood" (2002). These ominous words are followed by a montage of *noir* images over the sounds of thunder and lightning: full moon, howling wolf, dark stairs, candles, a cloaked figure, a woman's feet cautiously descending the staircase. An image of a nondescript dark-haired man in a cloak suddenly cuts to a close-up of the vampire's teeth; we hear growling and a woman's scream; and then we see the teeth biting into her neck and hear a sound of an animal tearing into the flesh of its victim. Sounds of loud gulping and a silenced heartbeat accompany the final image of teeth dripping with blood. Following these rather gruesome images, dawn arrives and a large cross appears, presumably on the grave of the vampire's victim, while the voiceover narration warns us of potential dangers of scientific discoveries: "As doctors begin to repeat and improve on Blundell's work, a terrible truth began to dawn on them. Transfusion of the human blood could just as easily kill as cure" (2002). This intertwining of vampire images with warnings about the dangers of blood transfusion sets up and informs the rest of the documentary. Though it assures us that Karl Landsteiner's 1901 discovery of blood types had "broken down the last barrier in the human quest to control blood," the documentary's ominous warnings transform the history and science of blood research into stories of angels and demons.

An illustrative example is the Nicaraguan blood scandal of the late 1970s. In 1977, the Nicaraguan dictator Anastasio Somoza Debayle and a Cuban exile, Dr. Pedro Ramos, opened a plasma center called "Plasmaferesis" in Managua. The center bought blood from the poor and the homeless. There were also reports that the government forced political prisoners to donate blood for the center. The blood was then sold to the U.S. and Western Europe. Pedro Chamorro, an editor of a leading oppositional newspaper called *La Prensa*, described Somoza's activities in print as an "inhuman trade in the blood of Nicaraguans." The National Red Cross, and other medical associations in Nicaragua, supported Chamorro's report. The plasma center became known as "The House of Vampires" and, with criticism growing, the Somoza government hired assassins to shoot down the editor on a street in January 1978. Riots and protests ensued with signs reading "Vampire Somoza!" The plasma center was burned to the ground. It is widely believed that this was a key incident in finally bringing Somoza's regime to an end (Kimbrell, 1993).

The documentary situates this event in the history of blood collection within the context of an increasing commercialization of blood and blood products. Douglas Starr sets the stage: "America was exporting more than anybody else. And Europeans were pretending that they didn't do it, although they were importing it and paying for it like crazy. And it came to the point where they had to find new sources for the material. Now the oil industry went to the Middle East and parts of Africa. But the question was, 'Where is the plasma? Where is the plasma cheap and plentiful and easy to get.' And it turns out the crowded cities of the Third World." Here he makes a parallel between blood and oil to indicate the scarcity of both resources. Tom Asher, the former division manager for Hyland Laboratories, then explains why Nicaragua developed the largest plasma donation center in the world: "They [poor Nicaraguans] were prized plasma donors for a variety of reasons. Their diets were infinitely better for producing plasma proteins. Beans and rice. They were great donors...obedient donors." (2002). While the documentary is critical of these practices, it mainly takes issue with how collecting "cheap" blood affected and polluted the Western body. Therefore, *Red Gold* weaves a complicated tale in which volunteer blood donation is seen as a remedy for corruption in a system that introduces the exotic, the poor and the contaminated Other into a civilized world of blood donation and community support.

In order to be considered dangerous, donors had to be rhetorically placed outside of civilized practices, whether sexual, cultural, or hygienic. For example, the final section of *Red Gold* shifts its attention to the exotic and dangerous Delhi, India. We are told that there is a blood shortage in India partially because blood is believed to be sacred and can only be given to gods in church rituals. Because blood donation policy in Indian hospitals requires that blood to be used for surgery be replaced in the blood bank before surgery can take place, and because paid donors are illegal, there are unofficial blood donors who stand by hospitals and make themselves available to impersonate a donating family member for a fee. The documentary warns that these donors may lie about their sexual and personal history. These cautionary tales are interspersed with vignettes of the "model" donor Paul Brown, whom I mentioned above. This contrasts the good, or implicitly moral, system with that which is dangerous and deceitful. Moreover, the narrator continues, bloodletting is still practiced on the streets of Delhi. The documentary shows us a lay healer who uses one razor blade for all clients; the story is told over exotic music and shots of overcrowded and dirty streets. It is unclear how many people take advantage of the healer's services, or the healer's status in the society, but the argument is clear. There are places in the world—unclean, overcrowded, dirty, dangerous places—that are out of step with rational Western science. The exotic and always racialized Others are implicated in the spread of diseases.

These tales would not be possible without a distinction between "blood" and "blood products." The Red Cross and other regional blood banks are nonprofit organizations that specialize in the collection of whole blood. Blood products, such as plasma and its derivatives (factor VIII, used for treatment of hemophilia, amongst others), are collected and processed by for-profit pharmaceutical companies. Since the collection of blood for blood products is much more complicated and time-consuming, the donors are almost always paid (Bayer, 1999). Thus the corporations are always looking for cheaper donor sources. That is why most plasma collection sites are located in poor neighborhoods. For example, the documentary describes a plasma center in Los Angeles located next door to liquor store. The center does not pay donors in cash, but rather in certificates redeemable at the liquor store.

The Food and Drug Administration (FDA) has been responsible for regulating blood and blood products since 1973. The "blood shield" policy instituted in the 1970s insisted that volunteerism had to replace whatever payment continued to exist for whole blood and to drive commercial blood from the market; amongst other measures, the FDA required all whole blood and its components to be labeled as derived from either "paid" or "volunteer" donors. This blood policy did not extend to plasma and its derivatives, presumably because plasma donors, as a rule, are financially compensated for their donations. However, the first public battle over the commercial status of blood began in 1962 with a historic legal case: *Community Blood Bank of the Kansas City Area, Inc. v. the Federal Trade Commission* (Kimbrell, 1993). The case asked whether blood or other body parts could be defined as commodities. In 1955 in Kansas a commercial blood bank, called the Midwest Blood Bank, had been set up. It was not a particularly savory operation. Situated in a Kansas City slum, it featured a sign reading "Cash for Blood." Many of its blood donors were described in the legal proceedings as "skidrow" types—the homeless and the mentally ill, alcoholics and drug addicts. Some critics referred to the bank as a "vampire" preying on these vulnerable individuals. Reportedly, the bank's operations were bizarre and unsanitary—"worms all over the floor," blood delivery in a beer can. The owners were reported to have no medical training or education. At the same time, the community that would supply blood from volunteer donors formed a nonprofit blood bank. It was called the Community Blood Bank of the Kansas City Area. Soon, doctors and hospitals entered into agreements to use Community Bank's blood as opposed to Midwest's blood. In 1962, Midwest filed a complaint with the FTC claiming that Community Bank was conspiring to put them out of business. In other words, here was a case of a commercial blood bank charging a nonprofit blood bank with creating a monopoly. In 1963, the FTC concluded that the defendants had conspired to restrain trade in the "commodity"of blood. The Community Bank appealed and maintained "blood was not a commodity for sale, [but] was a living human tissue used in a medical service" (Kimbrell, 1993, p. 13). Doctors testified that "blood could not be a 'product' because it is wholly made by the human body as a part of its own functioning; it was not manufactured for sale and consumption. They argued that calling blood a commodity was a dangerous "fiction" that would allow the market to be extended into other living parts of the human body" (Kimbrell, 1993, p. 14). In 1966, the FTC ruled on the case and sustained its original opinion that the Community Blood Bank and its cooperative hospitals, doctors, and others were guilty of conspiring to restrain Midwest Bank's trade in blood. The opinion argued that whole human blood could reasonably be defined as a biological product and thus the commercial banks are in the business of producing and selling a product. The appropriate monopoly laws would thus apply. In 1969 the Circuit Court reversed the FTC decision and declared that "nonprofit corporations without shares of capital, which are organized for and actually engaged in business for charitable purposes, and do not derive any 'profit'" (this included nonprofit blood banks), as outside of FTC jurisdiction (Kimbrell, 1993). While the decision did not comment on the nature of blood as a commodity, it allowed hospitals and healthcare professionals to use nonprofit banks freely without violating antitrust laws. Shortly after, the very idea of paid donors came under political and social scrutiny largely due to the rise of post-transfusion hepatitis infections and the publication in 1971 of *The Gift Relationship*. A controversial book by Richard Titmuss, a professor of social administration at the London School of Economics, *The Gift Relationship* passionately argues for an exclusive use of unpaid donors as a solution to the rising infection rates (1971).

In the 1960s, numerous studies started to suggest that the incidence of post-transfusion hepatitis has been higher in patients who have received transfusions of commercial blood than in those who have received transfusions of volunteer blood (Johnson 1977). Titmuss cited these multiple studies and argued that high rates of transfusion hepatitis in the United States can be attributed to its reliance on the commercial blood system:

> Under the standards set by the National Institute of Health, an ancient physician, a nurse and a former bartender can theoretically combine their resources to form a blood bank. They can draw most of their blood from Skid Row donors at the minimum fee and sell their blood to hospitals that seek the lowest bidder and are not concerned with the scientific aspects of blood banking. (p. 151)

Douglas Starr remarks in the documentary, "For Titmuss it was simple. Blood freely given was pure and clean. Blood that was paid for was not." Titmuss argued that there are reasons why paid donors were unsafe. First, he reasoned that skid row donors in need of money were more likely to lie about their health conditions than volunteer donors. He also argued that African American donors were more likely to provide inaccurate information about their health history:

> There is also the additional problem of examining and questioning coloured donors. These medical procedures applied to well-educated white donors (including questions about yellow jaundice) may produce reasonably accurate answers, but a coloured person, especially from a poor and unsophisticated background with inadequate

> medical knowledge and inadequate health services, could not be expected to know, for instance, whether or not he had had 'yellow jaundice," especially in his youth. The fact, therefore, that the whole of the United States blood donor program—and particularly the plasmapheresis program operated commercially with paid donors—relies to a substantial extent on supplies of blood from Negroes suggests that the risks of transmitted disease may be increased. (p. 152)

Here, on one hand, Titmuss is critical of medical institutions that exploit racial inequities and, elsewhere, is sensitive to how practices of blood segregation can contribute to a sense of alienation amongst racial groups (p. 71). On the other hand, he describes how an uneducated and unclean racial Other can contaminate the national blood supply. He assumes that African American donors are mostly paid donors who do not participate in the volunteer donation, or that categories of "whiteness" and "education," or as a matter of fact the category of "volunteer" itself, somehow ensures that donors will not be ignorant of their previous health conditions. Moreover, Titmuss's criticism of paid blood was not solely based on the danger of paid donors. To him, volunteer blood donation was an illustration of the moral altruistic gift relationship that was the fabric of society: "The forms and functions of giving embody moral, social, psychological, religious, legal and aesthetic ideas. They may reflect, sustain, strengthen, or loosen the cultural bonds of the group, large or small" (p. 71). For Titmuss, giving blood built and represented kinship, and he argued that in his study, most volunteer donors gave a moral reason for donating blood. He defines morality as a desire to contribute to society, an identification with a "universal stranger" whom the subject wants to help (p. 238). As Fontaine (2002) argues, at stake in Titmuss's argument was the reflection on what holds society together, as well as an implicit statement about the authenticity of morally based decisions. Economic motivations were not moral, and therefore not authentic. Fontaine writes that the dichotomy proposed by Titmuss between the social and the economic raises the question of the authenticity of social groups, bodies, and identities. For example, Titmuss writes, "Blood as a living tissue may now constitute in Western societies one of the ultimate tests of where the 'social' begins and the "economic" ends" (p. 18). In this view, the problem with paid donors is, in part, that economic selfishness underlies their decision to donate. I would add that it also implies that those who chose to become paid donors (skid-row donors, African American donors, prison donors) were outside of the universal kinship, and hence, outside of an underlying societal moral order. In other words, paid donors were dangerous to the very moral core of social relationships.

While critiqued for its condemnation of the commercial blood system in the United States and idealization of Britain's largely volunteer donor system (Hagen, 1982), *The Gift Relationship* had an enormous impact on the future discussion of blood policy (see Hagen, 1982; Hough, 1978; Johnson, 1977). As I mentioned above, Richard Nixon's secretary of health, education, and welfare put all blood donations under a system of federal control that labeled blood as either "volunteer donor" or "paid donor." In the 1970s, concerns about paid blood donation continued to grow, and in 1975, the Twenty-Eighth World Health Assembly of World Health Organization passed a resolution calling for non-paid donor systems to be set up in all member countries. The resolution shared Titmuss's assumption that paid blood, usually from the economically disadvantaged, was dangerous or impure (Glied, 1999). Those in the commercial blood business were perceived as guilty of spreading the diseases of disfranchised "Others," such as hepatitis, into the "normal" and "healthy" population. Less than a decade later, the HIV/AIDS pandemic brought new urgency to securing the safety of the blood supply, and the lines between Self and Other, "healthy" and "contaminated," "normal" and "deviant," became sharply drawn. In other words, blood donation has found its perfect articulation in HIV/AIDS.

I argued that blood is a boundary liquid that functions to demarcate difference and a powerful instrument for building community and identity. The *Red Gold* documentary creates a seamless narrative of community in which difference is managed through scientific and cultural exclusion and/or incorporation. In the process, certain struggles, sufferings, and deaths are assigned more gravitas than others. What emerges is a homogeneous account of a community that employs difference as a point of reference to itself: we do not have bad, tainted, evil blood and therefore we are good, innocent or righteous. And metaphors such as "bad blood" can only make sense if metaphors of blood as life first position blood as a totalizing entity that essentializes body and identity. The metaphor "blood is life" necessitates a narrative with its own heroes, victims, villains, and monsters. Of course, who gets to be a hero and who gets to be a monster is very much dependent on who is telling the story.

Mary Douglas (1966) writes:

> The body is a model which can stand for any bounded system. Its boundaries can represent any boundaries, which are threatened or precarious. The body is a complex structure. The functions of its different parts and their relations afford a source of symbols for other complex structures. We cannot possibly interpret rituals concerning excreta, breast milk, saliva and the rest unless we are prepared to see in the body

> a symbol of society and to see the power and dangers credited to social structure reproduced in small on the human body....Public rituals enacted on the human body are taken to express personal and private concerns....What is being carved in human flesh is an image of society." (pp. 116, 117)

And as an image of society is carved into human flesh, blood is bound to ooze out. Critical theory and cultural studies can provide a framework through which the body and blood can be understood as historically situated constructions that link popular culture and scientific discourse. These constructions inform both scientific practices and popular media, they educate and entertain, they attract and repulse. That is to say they tell us a story of what it means to be human and of what it *feels* like to occupy a body that inevitably leaks blood. And, as in any compelling story, there are heroes and villains, danger and suspense, monsters and humans. Moreover, blood becomes essential to storytelling associated with pandemics. In the next chapter, I turn attention to the HIV/AIDS pandemic, which demonstrates how narratives of blood inform moral panic informing the global parameters of the AIDS pandemic.

· 2 ·

HIV/AIDS AND MEDIATED NARRATIVES OF MORALITY AND CITIZENSHIP

Red Gold opens the section on the HIV/AIDS epidemic with the image of two men holding hands. A grave-sounding voiceover announces that the cultural exuberance about blood donations was dampened by a realization that "blood could be a deadly poison." While the documentary mainly discusses how the AIDS epidemic affected hemophiliacs and other patients who relied on blood and blood products, the establishing shot signifies that the dangers of HIV/AIDS are connected within the public imagination to the fears of possible contamination. As "an epidemic of signification" (Treichler, 1999), HIV/AIDS is a pandemic that produces various signifying practices that reinforce cultural categories of morality and danger. In this chapter, I analyze the HIV/AIDS pandemic in its various cultural contexts. Using theoretical approaches of moral panic, discursive formation, and citizenship, I argue that cultural representations of HIV/AIDS construct narratives of morality and citizenship as categories of inclusion and exclusion in civic life.

Theories of Moral Panic

Stanley Cohen (2002), in the book that introduced the concept of moral panic, describes a moment or a period of time when societies become subject to this phenomenon:

> A condition, episode, person or group of persons emerges to become defined as a threat to social values and interests; its nature is presented in a stylized and stereotypical fashion by the mass media; the moral barricades are manned by editors, bishops, politicians and other right-thinking people; socially accredited experts pronounce their diagnoses and solutions; ways of coping are evolved or (more often) resorted to; the condition then disappears, submerges or deteriorates and becomes more visible. Sometimes the subject of the panic is quite novel and at other times it is something which has been in existence long enough, but suddenly appears in the limelight. Sometimes the panic passes over and is forgotten, except in folklore and collective memory; at other times it has more serious and long-lasting repercussions and might produce such changes as those in legal and social policy or even in the way society conceives itself. (p. 9)

Cohen coins the term "folk devils" to describe those perceived to be responsible for the threat. For Cohen, the mass media is the most important agent to the development of the moral panic, especially in the early stages of producing images of deviants (Critcher, 2008; Hier, 2008). According to Cohen, the mass media "devote a great deal of space to deviance.…The media might leave behind a diffuse feeling of anxiety about the situation: 'something must be done about it'" (Cohen, 2002, p. 35). In this way, the media amplify deviance and thusly a corresponding moral panic. According to Critcher (2008), three processes are involved in the media's creation of moral panics: distortion or exaggeration, prediction of dire consequences, and finally, symbolization of words and images signifying threat. Cohen emphasized social psychological factors such as stress or anxiety—moral panics then became another form of social behavior (Thompson, 1998). As a result, moral panics orchestrate consent through an active intervention into the public opinion (McRobbie & Thornton, 1995). Cohen's analysis was criticized for its portrayal of society as monolithic and unchangeable, ignoring ideological power struggles inherent in constructions of deviance as a category (Critcher, 2008).

As Thompson (1998) points out, in order to become a moral panic, the threat must be aimed at the social order, including ideological and idealized dimensions. Moral panic then focuses on something more symbolic than the actual event itself. Hall, Critcher, Jefferson, Clarke & Roberts (1978) emphasized the ideological and hegemonic aspect of moral panics. Hier (2008) writes, "Hall et al. contend that the media serve as the primary means for disseminating moral panic but that the point of origin is to be found in processes of capital accumulation and 'crises in profitability.' Moreover, Hall et al. argue that in times of crises, the ruling elite 'orchestrate hegemony' by manipulating the media, which, in turn, reproduce structures and relations of domination"

(p. 177). For example, Hall et al. insist that a moral panic about muggings in 1970s Britain was a diversion from a crisis of capitalism. Moral panic therefore occurs when "the official reaction to a person, groups of persons or series of events is out of all proportion to the actual threat offered; it is when "experts," in the form of police chiefs, the judiciary, politicians, and editors perceive the threat in all but identical terms, and appear to talk "with one voice" of rates, diagnoses, prognoses, and solutions, when the media representations universally stress "sudden and dramatic" increases (in numbers involved or events) and "novelty," above and beyond that which a sober, realistic appraisal could sustain, that we then believe it is appropriate to speak of the beginnings of a moral panic" (Hall et al., [using "et al." for this entry going forward] 1978, p. 16).

Hall et al. draw on Gramsci's theory of hegemony, which states that dominant hegemonic regimes do not rule through direct oppression—although they do employ oppressive tactics when necessary—but rather by acquiring consent from the public (Gramsci, 2000). Therefore, the public sphere becomes a site where ideologies are negotiated, or a struggle for signification is deployed. Ideologies become dominant when they receive the consent of public opinion. Of course, this is not a purely democratic regime, and the dominant hegemonic regime maintains power through hedging debates to influence outcomes. However, the regime gains control and legitimacy through "winning" consent in these struggles. Hall et al. (1978) write, "The overall tendency is for the way the crisis has been ideologically constructed by the dominant ideologies to win consent in the media, and thus to constitute the substantive basis in 'reality' to which public opinion continually refers. In this way, by 'consenting' to the view of the crisis which has won credibility in the echelons of power, popular consciousness is also won to support to the measure of control and containment which this version of social reality entails" (p. 42).

Moral panic therefore is a manufactured site for ideological struggles and significations where "a 'silent majority' is won over to the support of increasingly coercive measure on the part of the state, and lends its legitimacy to a 'more than usual' exercise of control" (Hall et al., 1978, p. 42). The progressive escalation of threat necessary for moral panics is created through the "signification spiral," or "a self-amplifying sequence within the area of signification: the activity or event with which the signification deals is escalated—made to seem more threatening—within the discourse of signification itself" (p. 44). Convergence and thresholds help to escalate the signification spiral.

Convergence links two or more activities in the process of signification. For example, child kidnapping can be linked in a signification spiral with a failure of traditional community formation, and, in some cases, with fears of racialized "Others" (Thompson, 1998). Thresholds symbolically signify the limits of societal tolerance toward troubling events. For example, as I discuss later in the chapter, in the case of the AIDS pandemic, the threshold could be located at the point when HIV was transmitted via blood transfusions, thus enabling a symbolic signification of "innocent victims."

For Hall et al., the mass media is one of the most powerful forces in shaping of public consciousness and opinion. They write, "The signification of events in the media thus provides one key terrain where 'consent' is won or lost" (p. 41). Critcher (2008) reinterprets how Hall et al. see the role of media in constructing moral panic:

> First, the media are dependent on official sources of news, so act as secondary definers of such primary definers. Second, the media translate the statements of the powerful into a "public idiom," familiar to their readers. Third, the media feed back to primary definers their own reactions as if they were public opinion. Fourth, the media overemphasize violence in order to justify the extent of reaction. The result is a closed circle. (p. 1131)

The media are therefore a powerful force in maintaining a dominant hegemonic structure and in reinforcing dominant ideologies through an illusion of independent reporting and consent-building. The media do not consciously subvert public attention from economic problems, but rather economic problems put a strain on the media to which it responds by amplifying the symptoms, rather than causes, of the strain (Thompson, 1998).

The analysis of Hall et al. was criticized by numerous scholars for its portrayal of hegemonic institutions as having an absolute control over public opinion, saying that such a view ignored the role of countercultural movements in formation of cultural discourses (Hier, 2008; Stabile, 2001; Thompson, 1998). Moreover, McRobbie and Thornton (1995) argue that Hall et al. treat the media as a monolithic institution at the service of the elite. These critiques suggest that, as media become distributed across various platforms, a new theorization of moral panics must take into account oppositional cultural discourses produced by less traditional media.

Erich Goode and Nachman Ben-Yehuda (1994) build on Cohen's work and systemize the characteristics of moral panics using a social constructivist approach. They favor an interest-group approach to moral panic, inferring that moral panics are usually a result of middle-level rungs of power (Thompson, 1998). Goode and Ben-Yehuda argue that, often, moral panics serve the interests of a social movement or a group—for example the police or the media. In opposition to Hall et al., they argue that elites are marginal, and that "combined forces of grassroots feeling and middle-class agitation lie behind the most effective panics. The wider explanation lies in the nature of collective behaviour" (Critcher, 2008, p. 1133). Goode and Ben-Yehuda identify five elements or criteria of moral panic:

1. CONCERN—there must be a concern over the behavior and its consequences for the rest of the society;
2. HOSTILITY—there must be an increased level of hostility towards the "folk devils," "deviants," or those engaged in the threatening behavior, which "is seen as harmful or threatening to the values, interests, way of life, possibly the very existence, of the society, or a sizeable segment of that society" (p. 158);
3. CONSENSUS—there must be an agreement that the threat is "real, serious, and caused by the wrongdoing of group members and their behavior" (p. 158). According to Goode and Ben-Yehuda, while the consensus must be widespread, it does not need a majority in order to constitute a moral panic. Media can serve an instrumental role in representing a consensus about a threat. While a majority of people might not see a threat as serious, media representation can represent it as such through continuous and heightened coverage.
4. DISPROPORTIONALITY—concern must be out of proportion to the nature of the threat. Goode and Ben-Yehuda acknowledge that this criterion is hard to measure and ascertain. In response to this objection, they offer four indicators:

> First, if the figures that are cited to measure the scope of the problem are grossly exaggerated, we may say that the criterion of disproportionality has been met; second, if the threat that is feared is, by all available evidence, nonexistent, we may say that the criterion of disproportionality has been met; third, if the attention paid to a specific condition is vastly greater than that paid to another, and the threat or damage caused by the first is no greater than, or is less than, the second, the criterion of disproportionality may be said to have been met, and fourth, if the attention paid to a given condition at one point in time is vastly greater than that paid to it during a previous or later time without any corresponding increase in objective seriousness, then, once again, the criterion of disproportionality may be said to have been met. (p. 159)

5. VOLATILITY—moral panics are said to be volatile. Goode and Ben-Yehuda argue that while moral panics can vanish, or in turn be institutionalized or routinized, there is a "fever pitch" of moral anxiety and unrest, which does not last for a long time, but which is important to the functioning of moral panics.

Goode and Ben-Yehuda differ from Cohen in their perception of the role of the media in generating moral panic. In Cohen's analysis, the media are essential in the formation of moral panics: either as the prime movers or as a support system for those who are (Critcher, 2008). For Goode and Ben-Yehuda, the media are passive; they mainly serve as a conduit for middle-class anxieties (Critcher, 2008). Moreover, unlike Hall et al. (1978), they see the media as another middle-level interest group and do not connect it to the signification spiral or the perpetration of dominant ideologies (Thompson, 1998).

Moral Panic and Discursive Formation

The scholars discussed above employ structuralist approaches to assign particular categories of identification to the phenomenon of moral panic. They study how various institutional and ideological structures shape and represent moral panic, and while they disagree on particularities, they agree that the emergence of moral panics follows a linear path. This linearity aims to predict causes and effects of moral panics—an approach, however, that has been criticized by poststructuralist study of discourse and discourse formation. After all, moral panics are diffused and unpredictable—shaped as they are by numerous accidental forces. Critcher (2008) argues, "For the present purposes, the lesson is a disarmingly simple one: moral panics should be conceptualized as forms of discourse. Discourse analysis reveals how ways of speaking about an issue are constructed to subsume all other versions. Discursive formations prescribe who has the right to speak, on what terms and to which ends" (p. 1139). Therefore, current research uses the work of Michel Foucault, among other sources, to discuss moral panics as "discursive formations" where, "in particular times and places there emerge ways of speaking about social problems that assume dominance and privilege their terms and conditions over other" (Critcher, 2008, p. 1139).

The concept of discursive formation introduces discontinuity to the study of moral panics. Instead of continuous or linear history, Foucault (1972) urges his readers to focus on the present and the finite grouping of events, which constitute discourse about a topic at a particular point of time. This specificity focuses the subject of inquiry. Foucault remarks that "discourse must not be referred to the distant presence of the origin, but treated as and when it occurs" (p. 25). Instead of looking for underlying structures that explain everything about the world, Foucault (1972) argues that "the description of the events of discourse poses a quite different question: how is it that one particular statement appeared rather than another?" (p. 27) This means that, within a discursive formation, certain statements, or, for that matter, objects, emerge as being formative at a particular moment in time:

> Whenever one can describe, between a number of statements, such a system of dispersion, whenever, between objects, types of statements, concept, or thematic choices, one can define a regularity [or an order], we will say for the sake of convenience that we are dealing with a discursive formation....The conditions to which the elements of this division (objects, mode of statements, concepts, thematic choices) are subjected we shall call the rules of formation. The rules of formation are conditions of existence in a given discursive division. (p. 38)

Discursive relations form the objects of which they speak, or they "determine the group of relations that discourse must establish in order to speak of this or that object, in order to deal with them, name them, analyze them, classify them, explain them, etc." (Foucault, 1972, p. 46).

Discourse is then not a language, but instead a practice that forms and produces objects, knowledge, and statements of truth about a topic. Discourse does not simply restrict what can be said, but rather produces the multitude of ways in which we can talk and practice the subject of the discourse. For example, as I illustrate further in the chapter, the HIV/AIDS pandemic did not simply restrict sexual practices, but rather produced new categories of sexuality, which encouraged and discouraged certain types of sexual behavior. As scientific and cultural knowledge of HIV/AIDS expanded, so did its discursive formation—arguably, sex has never been talked about more. Thompson (1998) argues that Foucault's contribution to the study of moral panic could lie "in viewing controversies over various aspects of sexuality as signs of struggle over rival discourses and regulatory practices" (p. 25). In *The History of Sexuality Volume I*, Foucault (1978) argues that investment in human sexuality does not simply repress, but rather produces, manages, and classifies. If sexuality is a productive, not repressive, phenomenon, then we need to examine how discourse functions in relationship to sexuality, or what kind of knowledge is deemed authoritative, and what kind of pleasure is produced. Foucault writes:

> The central issue, then, is not to determine whether one says yes or no to sex, whether one formulates prohibitions or permissions, whether one asserts its importance or denies its effects, or whether one refines the words one uses to designate it; but to account for the fact that it is spoken about, to discover who does the speaking, the positions and view points from which they speak, the institutions which prompt people to speak about it and which store and distribute the things that are said. What is at issue, briefly, is the over-all "discursive fact," the way in which sex is 'put into discourse.'" (Foucault, 1978, p. 11)

The way in which sex is "put into discourse" is important for the discussion of the HIV/AIDS pandemic, either as a moral panic or as a discursive formation. How the media has put sex into the discourse of HIV/AIDS has shaped the moral panic associated with this pandemic.

HIV/AIDS, Moral Panic, and Discourse of Sexuality

A multiplicity of discourses surrounding HIV/AIDS does not lend itself to a singular cause and effect, while older models of moral panics do not sufficiently account for discursive formations of sex, pleasure, identity, and danger, all of which shape cultural response to the HIV/AIDS pandemic. Therefore, in order to analyze HIV/AIDS and the moral panics that it has created, we need to look at discursive formations of the disease. McRobbie and Thornton (1995) draw on the work of Simon Watney (1987):

> Classic moral panic theorists would ignore the daily endorsement (not to say enjoyment) of heterosexuality as an ideological norm and the consequences this has for those who are excluded. Policies and practices, which are concerned with "policing desire," do not, according to Watney, emanate from one or two centralized agencies of social control. They are endemic in media and society, and in this context the moral panic is best seen as a local intensification or "the site of the current front line" rather than a sudden, unpleasant and unanticipated development (Watney 1987:42)....Through considering the meanings which have developed around AIDS and homosexuality, Watney replaces the vocabulary of the moral panic with that of representation, discourse and the "other." (p. 565)

In fact Watney (1988) argues that a concept of moral panic cannot distinguish between different types of moral panic. Instead, we need to understand how moral panics can either draw on a single object of anxiety or serve as a diffused effect of multiple components. This is why, Watney (1987) argues:

> It is so important to avoid any temptation to think of the ongoing AIDS crisis as a form of "moral panic," which carries the implication that it is an entirely discrete phenomenon, distinct from other elements and dramas in the perpetual moral management of the home. On the contrary, homosexuality, understood by AIDS commentary as the "cause" of AIDS, is always available as a coercive and menacing category to entrench the institutions of family life and to prop up the profoundly unstable identities those institutions generate. The felt "problem" of sexual diversity is not established and imposed externally by the state, but rather internally, by the categorical imperatives of the modern organization of sexuality. (p. 76)

Even now, the AIDS pandemic is still a story of sexual and social mores. For example, cultural discourse draws sharp distinctions between its victims. There are "innocent" victims, and then there are those implicated in the acquisition of the disease through "risk behaviors." Jeffrey Weeks (1995) notes that at its beginning, AIDS was seen as a disease of "risk categories": "It was a disease that seemed to be confined to marginal, and politically and morally embarrassing, communities" (p. 79). He argues that, since 1982, AIDS "became the bearer of a number of political, social, and moral anxieties, whose origins lay elsewhere, but which were condensed into a crisis over AIDS" (p. 80). These "risk behaviors" became cultural representations of identities implicated in the disease. Identities were seen as "infected" prior to the pandemic, hence the disease was not something that happened to people, but rather a revelation of who they already were. On the other hand, "innocent" victims were portrayed in the media as heroes who were fighting an unfair disease. These were individuals who were infected not because of who they were, but because someone else's negligence caused an unforeseen contact with the tainted essence of the Other. Watney (1987) argues, "[P]eople misdescribed as 'AIDS carriers,' are widely understood to threaten the equally spurious unity of 'the family,' 'the nation,' and even 'the species'" (p. 76). The modern organization of sexuality, according to Watney, does not accommodate Cohen's description of folk devils. The "risk" subjects of the AIDS pandemic are not a speedily constructed identity used to generate the public's fear. Instead, they are multilayered representations—or "monstrous representations"—that betray more about social mores than they hide (Watney, 1987). DeYoung (1998) argues that "creation of such monstrous representations seems to be more of a process of pathologizing than demonizing" (p. 271). In this matter, AIDS is what

Treichler (1999) called an "epidemic of signification," which "produced a parallel epidemic of meanings, definitions, and attributions" (p. 315). Therefore, Treichler (1999) argues that the diversity of meanings produced by the AIDS pandemic has been difficult to manage, fix, or fully understand. The meaning of AIDS is always slipping—especially as we learn more about the disease. In this way, I argue, disease is best understood as a discursive formation rather than a fixed moral panic. As Gilman (2010) argues, "[C]onstructing diseases does not always mean inventing them. Often, real pathological experiences are rethought as part of a new pattern that can be then discerned, diagnosed, and treated. Illness and our sense of our own risk and our response to that risk shape how we experience the illness itself" (p. 1868). For example, the *Frontline* documentary "The Age of AIDS" (Barker, 2006), argues that "this is not just a disease, it's a social disorder that created all sort of reactions in society." The documentary also refers to HIV/AIDS as a "political problem" or a "political disease"—lending credence to the claim that HIV/AIDS is a pandemic of signification.

In 1982, the CDC established categorization of AIDS risk identities—the so-called "4H Club," which included homosexuals, heroin users, Haitians, and hemophiliacs. This classification shaped media portrayals of HIV/AIDS for decades to come. "The Age of AIDS" starts the story of AIDS in America with images of shirtless men dancing in disco clubs and a statement that the disease occurred in very large cities, which were the centers of "gay lifestyle". Dr. Jim Curran continues, "We were struck that all of the men were active gay men and were also struck that they had a complicated social lifestyle, involving a number of recreational drugs, as well as a large number of sexual partners. So it wasn't surprising that if a new infection were to come along, it could be focused in the gay community." The equation of sexual orientation with a particular lifestyle highlights HIV/AIDS as a disease of identity. What would be a lifestyle associated with heterosexuality? The documentary further exoticizes the disease through the portrayal of Haitian Americans who were dying of AIDS. It interjects the discussion of the epidemic in the Haitian community of Miami with shots of voodoo rituals, exotic chants, and healing practices. The focus on AIDS as the disease of the "4-H Club," and the subsequent media portrayals that emerge out of that description, had real-world consequences for treatment and prevention. It led to the exclusion of women from the diagnostic categories, which meant the misdiagnosis and death of thousands of patients (Treichler, 1999). However, even decades into the epidemic, it contributed to the spike of infection in the African American community, which did not see itself represented in the HIV/AIDS reports and narratives. The documentary "Endgame: AIDS in Black America" (Simone, 2012), discussed consequences of these representations:

> NARRATOR: When every patient with the new disease died, alarmed officials sent out an international alert. But from the start, something was missing.
>
> DR. MICHAEL GOTTLIEB: In medicine, when we describe a patient, we say, "This is a thirty-one-year-old white, single, gay male." But in our reports, we said nothing whatsoever about race. It really is an omission on our part.
>
> The first five patients were white. The next two were black. The sixth patient was a Haitian man. The seventh patient was a gay African American man, here in Los Angeles. Most of those first patients died within months. We had no information and treatment. In June of '81, we were thinking, "Oh, this is something among gay men here in Los Angeles. And yes, some are white and a couple are black. No big deal."
>
> NARRATOR: But it was a big deal. The media ran headlines of a killer plague among gay men. But the stories and the images were white.
>
> PHILL WILSON: I was a young, black, gay man from the south side of Chicago. I had never even heard of Fire Island. I was not a West Hollywood person. I had, you know, barely ever been—barely ever been to San Francisco. I was in San Francisco when I was ten years old. So none of this mattered to me. My thought was, you know, "Thank God it is them and not us. For once in a lifetime, it is about white people and it's not about black people."

Later on in "Endgame," a young African American woman describes how she never thought she was at risk for HIV/AIDS when she met her "Prince Charming":

> I remember in our wellness book, HIV was a picture of a helpless kid in Africa, and also a white, gay, skinny, skinny man.... In high school, I was most athletic. My best friend was prom queen. I was a heterosexual, not promiscuous, all-American teenager. I was, you know, just a normal girl. And just HIV and normal didn't go together, so I thought.... I wasn't shocked that I had contracted a virus that there was no cure for, one that was very hard to live with, I was shocked that I contracted a virus that I felt I would never get.

These examples illustrate material implications of discursive formations. How we talk about a disease impacts diagnosis and dissemination of a disease amongst a population. Another powerful example is the struggle for signification over definitions of guilt and innocence during the AIDS epidemic exemplified by mediated struggle between hemophiliac and gay communities.

AIDS and "Innocent" Victims

In its coverage of the AIDS pandemic, the *Red Gold* documentary uses a widely distributed story of Susie Quintana, known in the media as "Suzie Q." Described as an average woman living in the rural town of Dolores, Colorado, she accidentally shot herself with a rifle and needed a unit of blood. Her son asked about blood safety and was assured by the hospital that the blood was perfectly safe because "there were not any gays or homosexuals in the county." This was 1983 and Susie contracted HIV as a result of blood transfusion. While blood has always been pooled nationally, the documentary stipulates that the family did not know that Susie Q's blood did not come from inside the county, but rather from New Mexico. The donor was a gay man, who, the voiceover states, "thought he was safe because he was not promiscuous." In 1988 Susie became famous when she sued United Blood Service for giving her contaminated blood. In the early 1990s, on the day that she died, the Colorado Supreme Court ruled in *Quintana vs. United Blood Services* that the blood industry could be held negligent and awarded Susie's heirs a sum of eight million dollars (Bayer, 1999). This victory opened floodgates for massive litigation. Susie represented an "innocent" victim of AIDS who, according to the documentary, had "no other risk factors for HIV." Like other AIDS narratives, this case implied that people in rural towns do not engage in "risk" behaviors and that only those who engaged in such practices—even if these behaviors occurred in non-promiscuous relationships—can be implicated in the transmission and acquisition of AIDS. Such a dichotomy between dangerous/exotic "Others" and "innocent" victims framed much of the cultural experience of AIDS and became a powerful representation of the epidemic (Epstein, 1996; Fee & Fox, 1988; Kinsella, 1989, etc.). As such, it shaped the identities of its victims. Treichler (1999) writes, "Questions of identity involving who is infected and how HIV is transmitted shape fundamental understandings of what AIDS *is*; in turn, these understandings have shaped the ways we identify and classify those whom HIV infects as well as its modes of transmission" (p. 238).

The chronology of blood scandals during the AIDS epidemic illustrates the processes through which political and economical struggles over blood regulation became discursive struggles to define and maintain community boundaries in the face of an epidemic that crossed boundaries and drew an alliance in misfortune across various communities. For example, as the first hemophiliac was diagnosed with what was then known as GRID (Gay-Related Immune Deficiency) in June 1982, various hemophiliac groups decried the connection that was being made between GRID, immune suppression, and factor VIII. And in October of the same year, the National Hemophilia Foundation (NHF) adopted a resolution that urged "all sources of Factor VIII products to exclude from plasma donation individuals who were homosexual, intravenous drug users, or recent residents of Haiti" (Bayer, 1999).

The documentary talks at length about the devastation that HIV-infected batches of factor VIII caused to the hemophiliac community. Cory Dubin, a prominent hemophiliac activist, repeatedly refers to the "Hemophiliac Holocaust," a metaphor utilized to distinguish hemophiliacs from gay men and other unsavory or stigmatized victims of AIDS. In 1992, Michael Rosenberg organized the Hemophilia/HIV Peer Association, a militant activist group that issued a manifesto titled *Causes and Effects of the Hemophilia/AIDS Epidemic*, declaring "genocide" on grounds of the pharmaceutical companies' and the FDA's "reckless disregard" for this community's welfare. It stated that besides transfusion victims, hemophiliacs were the only people infected *because* they followed the advice of their doctors. It also condemned the NHF for initially advising hemophiliacs not to be alarmed by AIDS and called Dr. Louis Aledort, a leading medical adviser of the NHF, "The Mengele of the Hemophilia AIDS Holocaust" (Bayer, 1999). The distinction served well politically. In 1992 Congress appointed the Institute of Medicine (IOM) to undertake an inquiry into the blood industry's behavior during the first few years of the AIDS epidemic. The inquiry focused exclusively on hemophiliacs with no mention of the transfusion victims. The purpose of the committee was not to "assign blame," but rather to "objectively" describe the policy and science processes in order to provide policy developments to be pursued in the future effort to protect blood supply. Hemophilia activists expressed disappointment with the "tame" focus of the committee (Bayer, 1999; Shilts, 1988).

In 1993, numerous cultural discourses emerged to do away with the language of blood "services" and instead use the term "manufacturing industry." This is exemplified in the *Frontline* special "AIDS, Blood, and Politics" (Langer, 1993), a scorching indictment of the blood industry, as well as in the testimony of FDA commissioner Dr. David Kessler before a Congressional committee investigating the safety of blood supply. In the fall 1993, the IOM committee started its proceedings with testimonies of hemophiliacs who were living with AIDS, as well as families who had lost hemophiliac relatives to AIDS. They spoke of "murder" and demanded "justice." Again, no testimonies from transfusion AIDS victims were heard (Bayer, 1999). In 1993, the NHF attempted to seek a "financial assistance" program for hemophiliacs, and in 1995, the

IOM committee issued a report that many of the AIDS infections in those dependent on blood supply could have been avoided if the blood industry, doctors, and government institution had acted differently. However, it stressed the institutionally rooted inadequacy of the response as opposed to the moral failings that were emphasized by hemophilia activists. The committee urged the establishment of a new governmental position, the blood safety director. It further advised the creation of a no-fault compensation system for those who might suffer harm from blood or blood products in the future, but did not recommend a compensation system for those who are already HIV-positive (Bayer, 1999).

Finally, in 1998, the Ricky Ray Hemophilia Relief Fund was established to pay one billion dollars to an estimated eight thousand hemophiliacs and their infected spouses or surviving family members. Passed by a predominantly Republican Congress and supported by house speaker Newt Gingrich, the fund was designed to provide partial restitution for the failure of the government to secure the blood supply. First introduced and defeated in 1995, the proposal was not supported by the leading AIDS lobbying organization, the AIDS Action Council, whose members were offended by the implicit distinction between different kinds of AIDS victims (Bayer, 1999). The act was named after a fifteen-year-old boy who died from what the act calls "hemophilia associated with AIDS." Such wording of the cause of death, coupled together with the language of "responsibility" and "preventability," drew a distinction between hemophiliacs and other AIDS victims. While not all hemophilia organizations endorsed these distinctions, the *Red Gold* documentary does not problematize the implications of the Ricky Ray Act. For example, Cory Dubin comments: "It was a wonderful victory for the community. It was the community defending itself and going out for what is right."

Treichler (1999) also points out that media narratives of the HIV/AIDS pandemic often mix identity categories (gay men, hemophiliacs, heterosexual) with behavioral categories (IV drug user, transfusion patients). Thus, they mix risk groups with modes of exposure, thereby confusing "who you are" with "what you do." This is specifically illustrated in blood banks' guidelines, which require donors to indicate, not only if they are HIV-positive, but also if they are gay, or engaging in homosexual practices.

Gay organizations argued that these practices of donor screening resembled past blood laws that divided black blood from white blood, and could potentially lead to an event like the internment of Japanese Americans during WWII. Gay activists maintained that the quarantine of blood was an ominous first step towards further social, political, economic and even physical quarantine of a community already denied many basic civil rights protections. Stigmatizing the blood of an already disenfranchised segment of society could have permitted homophobic and racist forces to accomplish in the name of "science" what they thus far have been unable to fully accomplish politically. They argued that it is blood, not donors, which should be put to scrutiny, or, in other words, that blood needs to be separated from identities and bodies. However, in March 1983, the U.S. Public Health Service issued recommendations on the "Prevention of Acquired Immune Deficiency Syndrome," stating that due to a latency period between exposure and the onset of illness, physical examinations could not identify those with AIDS. Thus, there was no alternative but to exclude all members of groups at increased risk for AIDS. High-risk people include those gay men who were sexually active, had overt symptoms of immune deficiency, or had engaged in sexual relations with people who did. In January 1985 the Public Health Service further issued guidelines stating that all donors are to be informed that their blood will be tested for antibody to the virus and that they will be notified if the results are positive. Furthermore, those whose blood tests positive will be placed on the blood collection agency's donor deferral list. The FDA makes clear that blood testing is to serve *in addition* to donor self-deferral to close the "window" period of the disease. While gay organizations expressed concerns that deferral lists could be used to screen for "undesirables," the guidelines stuck. For political, economic, medical, and social reasons donors' identity remained metaphorically, symbolically, and irrevocably tied to their blood.

The gay organizations' references to the blood policy of the past draws a metaphorical connection between their experiences and those of people denied cultural citizenship because of their perceived blood alliances. These organizations are examples of people fighting to have blood treated as separate from a person's racial or sexual identity. These are not purely rhetorical debates. As I argued in the previous chapter, the debates over metaphorical meanings of blood have had material effects on persons' livelihoods and identities. They define and divide communities, construct "model" donor bodies, and determine who gets to participate in the community and on whose terms. They can also unite to create cohesive, unified, and seamless cultural narratives that show how bodies are constructed, managed, and understood through discourses of sexuality and disease. I would argue that these symbolic struggles are most entrenched within discourses of citizenship. The struggle of gay activists to be included in the blood supply was a struggle to be recognized as valid citizens of the United States. In fact, discursive associations between AIDS, a dangerous "Other," and citizenship are by no means unique to the United States. In Japan, there was also a widespread suspicion of foreigners as AIDS carriers. Public baths and massage parlors posted signs saying "No Westerners;" hostess clubs advertised "Japanese girls only" and "No foreign items work here." Popular sex nightclubs that featured foreign women closed due to the lack of customers. Even gay organizations emphasized Japanese ethnicity over sexual orientation, and safe sex often meant relations with other Japanese and the avoidance of "unsafe" foreigners, especially Westerners (Feldman, 1999). In the next section, I examine some of these myriad global discourses of AIDS and citizenship.

AIDS and Citizenship

In the previous chapter, I described how blood donation served as a narrative of nation building and what Jeffrey Bennett (2008) describes as a "performative act of civic engagement" (p. 6). A ritual of blood donation or sacrifice becomes associated, as Bennett argues, with a performance of citizenship, which interpolates its subject-citizens within a complex network of civic obligation and identity. As I have argued in the previous chapter, absorbed in the discourses of public health, such citizenship is connected to duties or responsibilities of "model" donors. Bennett (2008) makes that very point as well. "Health," he writes, "functions to reinforce mythic notions of the pure nation-state and the 'biological responsibilities' that accompany citizenship in that space" (p. 13). Here, citizenship becomes an imaginary discourse, connecting the private bodies of its citizens to a larger social body of the nation-state. Lauren Berlant (1997) explains:

> Once it is established that national culture demands a continuous pedagogical project for making people into "private citizens" who understand their privacy to be a mirror and a source of nationality itself, it becomes equally important that the national culture industry generated a mode of political discourse in which the nation form trumps all other images of collective sociality and power. (p. 56)

Once a link between "private citizen" bodies and the health of the nation-state is established, the threat to one becomes a matter of national security for another. The representation of the spread of HIV/AIDS in "The Age of AIDS" emphasizes the connection between disease and national security. The documentary makes a connection between destabilized government regimes and the rise of the pandemic, especially in cases of Russia and South Africa, where the fall of communism and apartheid respectively coincided with the rising rates of HIV/AIDS. In Russia, the documentary ascribes the rise of HIV/AIDS to government destabilization: "In Russia, the end of communism brought cheap heroin—and AIDS.…Along busy highways, some drug users paid for their habit with sex.…Businessmen…Men carried the virus home to their families. Soon nearly one million Russians were infected. In Moscow, the government did almost nothing" (Barker, 2006).

The documentary also stresses a connection between HIV/AIDS, globalization, and an increasing ease of movement across national borders: "In the age of globalization, HIV thrived. Following sex and the drug trade, it spread across Eastern Europe, through Southeast Asia into India and China, the most populous countries on the planet." According to the documentary, Chinese response to HIV/AIDS was driven by a realization that their "closed" society was not a match against forces of globalization. A special session of the Security Council on AIDS reasserted those fears. The documentary stresses this point:

> RICHARD HOLBROOKE, U.N. Ambassador, Clinton Administration: I came up with the idea that we should hold a special session of the Security Council on HIV/AIDS. I was told by everyone, including my own staff, "You can't do this. It's not done. It's not in the UN Charter." And I said, "But AIDS is a security issue because it's destroying the security, the stability of countries."
>
> Vice President AL GORE: I call to order this first meeting of the United Nations Security Council in the twenty-first century. When ten people in Sub-Saharan Africa are infected every minute, when eleven million children have already died… when a single disease threatens everything from economic strength to peacekeeping.

Throughout its investigation into the origins of HIV, "The Age of AIDS" stresses narratives of citizenship, national security, and globalization. As with most Western media coverage of the HIV/AIDS pandemic, the documentary mostly cares about the spread of the disease into the United States and Europe. This implies that a disease only becomes a problem when it travels into the developed world. The documentary engages in an argument amongst government officials and doctors who are wary of media coverage, but, at the same time, reinforce stories of dangerous, exotic people who can take infection from one continent to another.

> DR. JOSEPH B. McCORMICK, M.D., CDC, 1974–93: We now know, based on the advanced symptoms that we say, that this disease had been circulating for quite a while. And therefore, we had to understand better where it might have come from, and in particular, where did it go. Somehow, the disease had gotten into the U.S. and Europe. And so the question is, "Well, who would have been at risk and could have taken the disease out of the Congo?" There were a few choices: Europeans living there, Belgians primarily, but French and others, and Congolese who were leaving the country to go abroad and Haitians.
>
> NARRATOR: When independence came to the former Belgian Congo and the Europeans left, the new government contracted with Haiti to bring French-speaking professionals—teachers, nurses and doctors—to fill the jobs left behind....Haiti, one of the poorest countries in the world, would prove to have few defenses against the disease. It was in the late '70s and early '80s that local doctors noticed that more and more young Haitians were coming to them or seeking healing spells from a local priest for a new wasting disease....In one of the roughest parts of Port-au-Prince, Dr. Jean Pape started the first AIDS clinic in Haiti. Yet Dr. Jean Pape was convinced the disease had been first brought to the island by homosexual tourists from America.
>
> DR. JEAN PAPE: Haiti was a haven for homosexuals because sex with a male Haitian was very cheap. They didn't call themselves homosexuals because the same Haitians would also have contact with many more women.
>
> NARRATOR: It was also a time when thousands of Haitians were fleeing the island's poverty and corruption. The U.S. media were doing stories about "boat people." And now there were reports of sick Haitians showing up in Dr. Margaret Fischl's hospital in Miami.
>
> DR. MARGARET FISCHL: One of the local channels called me up and was almost whispering on the phone, said, "Is it true Haitians brought in a deadly disease in the United States?" And I said, "That better not be your headline in tomorrow's paper."
>
> NARRATOR: But those were the headlines when the CDC sent out a warning to physicians about the reports of Haitian immigrants with the disease. In the press, it became a label—Haitians were a risk group.

This is a theme to which I return throughout the book, because pandemics are often a site of culturally drawn distinctions between individual, national, and global. Focus on citizenship as a discursive category focused on constructing citizenship underscores limitations of moral panic theory for the global HIV/AIDS pandemic.

For example, Berkman, Garcia, Muñoz-Laboy, Miguel, & Parker (2005) argue that categories of "citizenship" and "solidarity" were essential to the

Brazilian response to HIV/AIDS, where citizenship defined the relationship between the people and the state. Brazil's halt of HIV/AIDS infection is widely viewed of one of the success stories in the developing world. While infection rates skyrocketed as high as 25 percent in South Africa, Brazil's infection rate has remained at 1 percent. These results are largely due to Brazil's decision to break patents in order to manufacture anti-AIDS drugs (BBC News, 2004). Brazil's government based this decision on the WHO rule that allows a nation to break drug patents during a national emergency. Local activists, in alliance with international organizations, politicized drug patents as a matter of fair global exchange and social justice (Biehl, 2004). Biehl (2004) writes:

> As AIDS has officially become a matter of international security...Brazil has championed the autonomy of nations to break intellectual property rights in the name of securing its citizenry's health....This late-born democratic practice of citizenship through patienthood (or at least a claim to it) would transform in the subsequent years (and at an impressive speed) into a focused and sophisticated practice of care for one's pharmaceutical well-being. These individuals and their AIDS community would become less confrontational with political forces, local and national, less absorptive of street life, and more integrated with the life-guaranteeing mechanisms and technologies associated with the AIDS program, local and national. (pp. 108, 121)

In fact, Brazil's successful prevention campaign frequently utilized discourses of citizenship and equality. A 1997–1999 media campaign used the following slogans:

> *Do you know what happens when a friend of yours gets the AIDS virus? He keeps on being a friend of yours. Equality is the best treatment.*
> *Citizenship: An efficient weapon against HIV.*
> *Prevention begins with a dialogue. Discuss it, learn and live without AIDS.*

Instead of disfranchising, or excluding affected and infected groups, Brazil's prevention efforts incorporated them into a national conversation and made them useful citizens in the fight against the disease. Groups that are usually socially vulnerable, such as gay men and sex workers, developed a strong public voice in the dispute over access to public and medical resources (Biehl, 2004). This approach led to morality-based conflicts with the developed world and particularly with the 2003 U.S. fifteen-billion-dollar program known as the President's Emergency Plan for AIDS Relief, which required potential beneficiaries to make an explicit statement of policy opposing prostitution and sex trafficking (Rohter, 2005). This posed a problem for Brazil, where prostitution is not illegal and sex workers actively work with AIDS prevention groups. As a *New York Times* article reports:

> The Brazilian program very early on attempted to recognize that this is a pandemic that could travel through the population if there weren't programs to provide education and give special attention to vulnerable groups," said Mark Schneider, who was the Agency for International Development's director for Latin America in the Clinton administration and has worked at the Pan-American Health Organization. They attempted to take out the stigma and practice safe sex so as to prevent the epidemic from expanding, and in that way they were well ahead of other countries, particularly in the developing world. But the Brazilian approach is anathema to many conservatives in the United States because it makes use of methods seen as morally objectionable. Brazil not only operates a needle and syringe exchange program for drug addicts but also rejects the Bush administration's emphasis on abstinence, being faithful and the controlled use of condoms, the so-called ABC approach, in favor of a pragmatism that recognizes that sexual desire can sometimes overwhelm reason. (Rohter, 2005)

As a result of these restrictions, Brazil turned down forty million dollars in U.S. aid. Narratives of citizenship deployed by the Brazilian government to fight the epidemic were too important to forsake for international money.

While Brazil's prevention programs embraced its culture's public openness about sexuality, in Thailand the state was challenged to move sexual practices from the private sphere into the public arena (Fordham, 2001). As a result, it became one of the most effective governments in the region in controlling the course of the epidemic (Erni, 2006). The media prevention campaigns asked "good" Thais to have a blood test prior to having a baby (Fordham, 2001, p. 272). Indeed, in their media prevention campaigns, the Thai government deployed citizenship tropes to portray HIV/AIDS as an existential threat to the very existence of Thai people. For example, one TV spot showed black-and-white photo portraits slowly turning red one by one. Over ominous chorus music, a sinister male voice proclaimed: "It is a dangerous epidemic that's spreading fast. If we don't stop HIV now, in ten years there may be no Thai people left" (*AIDS in Thailand*, 2005). Thai media campaigns had a foreboding tone, but they served to combat a widespread belief that HIV was a foreign disease and would not become a national problem (Barker, 2006). Prevention campaigns spearheaded by senator and AIDS tsar Mechai Viravaidya—known in Thailand as "Mr. Condom"—were focused on condom distribution, sex education, and on a connection of HIV/AIDS prevention to a nationalist sentiment. For example, Viravaidya opened a chain of restaurants called "Cabbage and Condoms" to associate condoms with a national food staple (Barker, 2006). The prevention efforts worked—Thailand is a regional leader in the fight against HIV/AIDS.

In contrast to Brazil and Thailand, Cuba's HIV/AIDS prevention program did not garner international acclaim despite its success in controlling the epidemic. Cuba's initial response to the disease was to socially isolate infected individuals in sanatoria (Scheper-Hughes, 1993). Conditions at sanatoria were humane: patients were still receiving full-time salaries from their employers, could practice their trade (when possible) from the sanatorium, had access to amenities not widely available to the general population (such as color TVs), and gay men were able to openly have relationships with each other (McNeil, 2012; Scheper-Hughes, 1993; Swanson, Gill, Wald, & Swanson, 1995). Scheper-Hughes (1993) summarizes the rights and responsibilities of patients at sanatoria as follows: "Every patient has to respect the three 'commandments' of the sanatorium: (1) to have unprotected sex with an unknowing, uninfected individual is murder; (2) to have unsafe, but consensual sex, with an uninfected partner is criminal; and (3) to have unprotected sex with another infected partner is mutual suicide. Safe sex is the right of every resident, and there is no policing of sexual activity. 'We do not follow residents into their bedrooms,' the medical director told me. The surveillance is indirect and largely epidemiological" (p. 47).

The response from the international community was largely scornful. As a *New York Times* article states, Dr. Jonathan Mann, the first AIDS director at WHO, called them "pretty prisons" (McNeil, 2012). Scheper-Hughes (1993) writes, "The Cuban AIDS program has been criticized for its violation of the privacy and freedom of seropositive people. Most of the criticism has focused on the isolation of people in sanatoria....Cuban health officials remain uncowed by criticism: Cubans, they say, are not dying of AIDS. The international community remains unimpressed: in place of the aphorism 'the operation was a (technical) success but the patient died' one hears it said that Cubans may not be dying of AIDS but the operation is a (moral) failure" (p. 46). Cubans, however, were largely willing to follow the program, and even those confined to a sanatorium philosophically acknowledged its necessity. For example, in an interview with *60 Minutes*, one of the patients is asked if he is angry about having to leave his kids to live with relatives. He contemplates that "yes, on one hand I can be angry about that, but on the other, I am sick so I have to be here" (How Cuba Deals with AIDS, 2013). Swanson et al. (1995) argue that "Cuba's AIDS program is focused on promoting the common good by protecting the population from exposure to the HIV virus and providing comprehensive care for persons who have been infected with HIV or diagnosed with AIDS.…The willingness of the HIV-infected Cuban people to agree to Cuba's policy is supported by the basic underlying philosophy of subordination of individual desires to the common good. This personal sacrifice…meets the needs of the nation" (pp. 33, 39). The restrictions on outside visits eased in 1989 when trusted patients could leave, and, in 1993, the gates were opened as Cuba transitioned to largely outpatient care, with only three sanatoria remaining for those needing in-patient care (McNeil, 2012). The sanatoria did work for controlling and dampening the epidemic, however, despite the moral aspersions cast by the international community. More importantly, Cuban sanatoria, together with prevention programs in Brazil and Thailand, demonstrate how discourses of citizenship shape the responses to and the experiences of a pandemic. In fact, a successful appeal to citizen identity in the prevention campaigns can have a vast effect on the course of a pandemic. In the next section, I examine how similar narratives of citizenship and communities shaped Africa's response to the pandemic, albeit a much less successful one.

AIDS and Africa

As was argued above, the AIDS pandemic illustrates how cultural narratives shape the disease as a threat to national and global security. Bennett (2008) writes:

> The expansiveness of AIDS has given rise to a new set of complications for communal conceptions of citizenship and the role of the individual in the body politic.… AIDS has signaled the loss of the body, the implosion of identity, and the stagnation of development.…The apocalyptic implosion of the citizen subject signals a loss of bio-political control and the reproduction of civic actors and sacrificial bodies.…In the cultural imaginary AIDS is still largely conceived as prompting disintegration.… National discourses not only distance the threat of AIDS as a foreign entity rhetorically, they also seek to establish the idea that AIDS can be subsumed by invoking laws that speciously claim to protect the nation's boundaries. (pp. 43, 44)

According to Priscilla Wald, media representations distinguished between dangerous exotic "Others" and "model" healthy citizens, as risk groups became the enemy within (2008). In the meantime, in the media, the heterosexual face of the HIV/AIDS pandemic was displaced to Africa—an "impure" continent where the threat of the disease was directly linked to supposedly barbaric sexual practices. This displacement, according to Bennett, allowed for a recuperation of the normative heterosexual citizenship. He writes, "Displacing heterosexual AIDS to another continent has alleviated fears among heterosexual practices that seemingly do not implicate their identities" (p. 44). As Wald (2008) argues, even at the beginning of the AIDS pandemic, the search for the mythic Patient Zero—supposedly a French Canadian flight attendant—became rapidly Africanized in the mainstream media through speculations of sexual contact with Africans. Images of African primates deployed by numerous HIV/AIDS news stories at the onset of the pandemic did much to cement the African nature of the AIDS pandemic. In fact, "The Age of AIDS" begins with images of African forests and sounds of hollering monkeys. Wald (2008) writes, "As accounts of African AIDS conformed to familiar narratives, the metaphor of the Third World slid into a threat, and geographical boundaries were recast in temporal terms" (p. 237), while Erni (2006) writes, "The political realities of the global AIDS crisis are in many significant ways a direct mirror image of the geopolitical realities of 'Third World' postcolonial development" (p. 431). These geopolitical realities have in turn shaped Western narratives of HIV/AIDS in Africa. These narratives have included tropes and characters based in Western cultural assumptions about Africa as a continent. Austin (1989) identifies the cast of characters within the "AIDS in Africa" narrative:

> The Black subject takes the form of four central characters: one, the philandering urban male; two, the female prostitute; three, the victimized wife; and four, the male homosexual….Simultaneous with the notion of the Prostitute as the source of AIDS is a second origin story. Africa is established as the original site of production of the virus, generated from the depths of the jungle: "[Scientists are looking for an] AIDS-causing virus in baboons, chimps and green monkeys found in Central Africa, because epidemiologists suspect that the human AIDS epidemic originated in that part of the world." Although in some ways the stories seem to arrive at dissimilar conclusions, they function more to reinforce rather than to contradict each other. It is through the Prostitute that Africa becomes the motherland of AIDS. At this juncture in the search for the origin of AIDS, the role of the Prostitute and of Africa are conflated. (pp. 132, 135)

"The Age of AIDS" demonstrates a conflation of prostitution, the origin of AIDS, and Africa. Starting at the Congo Basin—illustrated once more with images of the forest and sounds of African drums—the documentary asserts that the virus came from a chimp somewhere in central Africa. Over gruesome shots of butchered chimpanzee parts, including severed heads, the narrator states that "hunting and butchering a chimpanzee would almost certainly involve blood-to-blood contact" (2006). The documentary continues:

> BEATRICE HAHN, M.D., University of Alabama: It is not known what has to occur for a newly transmitted chimpanzee virus to then become an epidemically spreading pathogen. There are a number of speculations that people have been putting forward which are quite reasonable and have to do with the basic biology of this virus, as we understand it today. Those speculations are increased partner change, if this person who has the chimpanzee virus gets introduced into a population with sexual promiscuity.
>
> DON FRANCIS, M.D., CDC, 1972–92: What happened in Africa is the urbanization of Africa, so where instead of living in the bush, that one now, especially males, migrated to the urban centers for work. Now the infected chimpanzee butcher comes into a larger city in Africa, now has sex with a woman, who has sex with a lot of other people. And now the woman gets infected, and thousands of other people get infected. And then it goes on and on and on. And this virus just searches out, and when there's an amplification system, it takes off.

Here an assumption of promiscuity is placed both on the population of Africa and on the body of a woman: the chimp butcher is not described as promiscuous, but a woman is. The narrative is repeated in the documentary's description of Uganda: "The long-distance drivers who traveled from the Kenyan coast of Mombasa on their way to Congo, Burundi, and Rwanda, used to stay there overnight. And therefore, it became popular with commercial sex workers. And the nightlife was very lively. It was nonstop happiness, later to turn into misery" (2006).

Western media coverage of Africa and AIDS implicates a "good time" girl in the spread of the disease, while projecting assumptions of prostitution and promiscuity onto the entire continent. Sacks (1996) argues that AIDS discourses about women, especially in Africa, focus on a figure of a prostitute as a polluter, which "concerns assumptions about prostitution as a dangerous form of female pollution, and prostitutes as a category of persons especially likely to be diseased and contagious" (p. 61). As a consequence, she argues, these discourses reverse the actual power relationships between male clients and female prostitutes. Moreover, these portrayals are intimately connected to discourses of citizenship—whose bodies are going to count and whose bodies are going be held responsible. As Sacks writes, "Another important theme in U.S. culture that is implicit in AIDS discourses about both prostitutes and HIV-positive mothers is that of self-control and self-discipline. AIDS discourses imply that HIV can be prevented through disciplined behavior, and that therefore those who become infected with it are responsible for their illness. In the context of AIDS, 'promiscuous' or 'indiscriminate' sex as well as IV-drug addiction or 'inappropriate' pregnancy, become powerful indices for loss of control. The properly disciplined body uses sex and intoxicants in controlled and socially acceptable ways" (p. 69). Narratives such as this, which connect promiscuity and Africa, are repeated throughout Western media. A *New York Times* article from 1990 openly wonders, "No one knows if Africans are more sexually active than people elsewhere. Adultery and short-term hotels can be found around the world, and some researchers wonder if Africans are any more promiscuous than, say, the sexually active populations of American cities.…Many researchers regard today's sexual behavior largely as a cultural aberration brought on by colonialism, urbanization and other recent trends. But others see it also as a pattern rooted in Africa's agricultural past and its tradition of polygamy" (Tierney, 1990).

In many ways, the story of AIDS in Africa is the story of women's bodies. Even Africa itself is represented as a woman—a continent in need of control, help, and discipline from the paternal West, while within Africa's own prevention efforts, HIV/AIDS is seen as a consequence of cultural departure from strong community values as evidenced by proliferation of fatherless families, and grandmother-headed households (Kaarsholm, 2005; Stadler, 2003). Moreover, Stadler (2003) writes, "[V]illagers believe that male and female blood is mixed and exchanged during sexual intercourse and that menstruation cleanses the body of accumulated 'dirty blood'.…At certain times (death in the family, menstruation), blood is polluting and sexual restraint is required to limit its transmission. Elders explained that the severity of the AIDS epidemic in the current setting is caused by the widespread failure to observe the rules of sexual behavior (milawu)" (p. 362). Therefore the burden of maintaining values and traditions falls onto women. For example, Kaarsholm (2005) describes the virginity tests in KwaZulu-Natal—a province of South Africa:

> The second, more prosaic variety of virginity testing—with a more toned-down and "hygienic" discourse—is illustrated by an interview held with Mrs Jane Chiwambere Phewa (the wife of councillor Phewa) and a group of Amaoti "health volunteers" in 1999. The goal of the volunteers is "to try to stop AIDS from escalating," and they believe that the prospect of virginity testing will help in making young girls abstain from sexual relations. Also "keeping track of virginities" will assist in bringing early attention to cases of rape inside or outside of families, which are seen by the group to be a major problem. As to culture, "the more we talk about it and do it, the more we may get into culture," but this is a long-term perspective, and the basic effort is a

> "technical" one of monitoring and controlling girls' sexual behaviour. As to questions of human rights infringements, Mrs Phewa sees this only from the parents' point of view: "we are not forcing anybody to let their children undergo this process, it is a choice inasmuch as she or he accepts that his or her child should undergo the virginity test—it is up to them. It is not something we force on people." (p. 149)

In the Western media, the HIV/AIDS pandemic in Africa has been mainly connected to women's bodies. Both *Newsweek* and *Time* ran stories on AIDS in Africa featuring a prominent picture—and, in case of *Time*, a cover picture—of an African woman holding a child (*Newsweek*, January 17, 2000; *Time*, February 12, 2001). Sacks (1996) writes that such images communicate "good" mother discourses, where

> HIV-positive women, in addition to being whiter in discourses than they are in hospital beds, almost always appear in the context of their children—and these children are the overwhelming, if not total, focus of such depictions. For instance, in the articles referred to above on women's experiences with AIDS, nearly all the women depicted either had grown sons with HIV, or were HIV-positive themselves and had HIV-positive children. While women's concern about what will happen to their children is natural, such women's exclusive concern with this issue seems less so. Notions of "good" or "bad" mothers come into play in this context. Those women sympathetically portrayed are often depicted as preoccupied over what will happen to their children after they die—a preoccupation that seems to obliterate any concern about their own fate. "Good" HIV-positive mothers, then, are characterized by self-denigration for having transmitted the virus to their children, and by selflessness regarding their own fates. Such depictions, while sympathetic in some respects, are nonetheless one-sided. (p. 68)

These depictions emphasize a connection between women and children—the child being the true "innocent" face of AIDS. Media narratives of AIDS in Africa acquire their true pathos when cases of children dying of AIDS are described. *Newsweek* and *Time* tell chilling stories of orphaned children abandoned by their relatives and communities; of dying three-year-olds and their infected mothers; and of teenage girls turned to prostitution. These stories portray Africa as a completely devastated continent incapable of taking care of itself. A *Time* cover story states:

> As the HIV virus sweeps mercilessly through these lands—the fiercest trial Africa has yet endured—a few try to address the terrible depredation. The rest of society looks away. Flesh and muscle melt from the bones of the sick in packed hospital wards and lonely bush kraals. Corpses stack up in morgues until those on top crush the identity

> from the faces underneath. Raw earth mounds scar the landscape, grave after grave without name or number. Bereft children grieve for parents lost in their prime, for siblings scattered to the winds. (Mcgeary, 2001)

The implication behind these stories is that only the West can save Africa from herself. Much like narratives of women, stories of Africa deprive the continent of its agency—be it political, social, or economic. It is instead a rescue mission of a continent incapable of taking care of itself. *Time* continues:

> AIDS in Africa bears little resemblance to the American epidemic, limited to specific high-risk groups and brought under control through intensive education, vigorous political action and expensive drug therapy. Here the disease has bred a Darwinian perversion. Society's fittest, not its frailest, are the ones who die—adults spirited away, leaving the old and the children behind. You cannot define risk groups: everyone who is sexually active is at risk. Babies too, unwittingly infected by mothers. Barely a single family remains untouched. Most do not know how or when they caught the virus, many never know they have it, many who do know don't tell anyone as they lie dying. Africa can provide no treatment for those with AIDS. (Mcgeary, 2001)

Of course, this portrayal of an African pandemic implies that the United States, as an affluent and "civilized" country, is able to protect its citizens. This is, of course, not the case. HIV/AIDS treatment in the United States is a privilege of those who can afford medications or have good health insurance. There is also a racial reality of the disease. In fact, the disease devastates African American communities in the United States. From the documentary "Endgame" (Simone, 2012):

> BAMBI GADDIST, Ph.D., South Carolina AIDS Coalition: I believe we should make an investment in other countries, but I also know that I'm in Africa right now. As a state, I'm there. Sometimes my staff feels like we're there. Every time we test another young person positive, we're there. The question is, "What is in the best interest of our community?"
>
> NARRATOR: At home in the U.S., there were places where the lifesaving new medicines were a long time coming, especially in the South, in places like Selma, Alabama.
>
> PHILL WILSON: When you look at the AIDS epidemic in Black America and you think about Black America as if it were a country unto itself, it would have the sixteenth worst AIDS epidemic in the world. If Black America were a country unto itself, it would be eligible for PEPFAR dollars.

In order to address these health disparities, we have to address HIV/AIDS as a global pandemic of inequality. Media narratives, however, do not allow for radical political interpretations of the disease. Instead, through discursive processes of identification and naming, the media individualizes the virus, and it obtains an identity of its own—as an alien killer of blood cells. "The Age of AIDS" documentary represents HIV as an intelligent, *conscious*, and self-aware enemy: "HIV has figured how to hide most of its surface behind sugar. Sugar is not foreign so our immune system cannot find it. The proteins—the foreign part of HIV—are hidden behind sugar so our bodies cannot find any crevice in this virus that it can attack and kill. HIV is amazing in the number of ways in which it can protect itself against our immune defenses" (2006). Viscerally illustrating this understanding of HIV/AIDS, a *Time* magazine cover magnifies an image of "HIV attacking a healthy T-cell" to emphasize the monstrous representation of the virus as a grey, tentacled, alien creature (*Time*, August 12, 1985).

In these representations, blood cells are presumed to be healthy prior to viral invasion and the internal struggle between the virus and healthy blood cells is mapped onto the external struggle to keep bodies and communities safe from contact with dangerous, alien, and presumably tainted Others. Metaphors of tainted blood become metaphors of tainted communities. Susan Sontag (1989) writes about how metaphors of war, invasion, and enemy have shaped the virus's identity:

> AIDS has a dual metaphoric genealogy. As a microprocess, it is described as cancer is: an invasion. When the focus is transmission of the disease, an older metaphor, reminiscent of syphilis, is invoked: pollution. (One gets it from the blood or sexual fluids of infected people or from contaminated blood products). But the military metaphors used to describe AIDS have a somewhat different focus from those used in describing cancer. With cancer, the metaphor scants the issue of causality....In the description of AIDS the enemy is what causes the disease, an infectious agent that comes from the outside....In the era of Star Wars and Space Invaders, AIDS has proved an ideally comprehensible illness. (pp. 105–106)

These metaphors and narratives ignore the systematic inequalities, injustices, and prejudices which have existed in communities and nations prior to the disease and which shape and determine social, medical, and political responses to the pandemic. Therefore, we must be wary of individualizing discourse, which alienates the disease and the bodies it afflicts from the larger geopolitical context in which they exist.

· 3 ·

VAMPIRES AND HIV/AIDS IN THE POPULAR IMAGINATION

The film *Near Dark* (Feldman, Nabatoff & Bigelow, 1987) tells a story of an all-American young man named Caleb who, along with his father, runs a ranch somewhere in the American heartland. One day he meets a beautiful woman named Mae in a local bar. He gives her a ride in his truck, and, during a kiss, she bites his neck and leaves behind puncture wounds. Mae runs away and Caleb chases her. But as the sun rises, he starts having trouble walking. He becomes sweaty, pale, and sick. He tries to stumble home, but a white van appears on the road and he is dragged inside. He is now a part of Mae's family: a gang of violent thugs who enjoy picking fights and killing people. They are, of course, vampires. The word "vampire", however, is never mentioned and, because it does not directly reference the supernatural, the film functions predominantly as a Western outlaw tale. The gang likes to drink their victims' blood, but they cut their throats with knives, and blood consumption can be seen as a psychotic, but human, ritual. There are no historical expositions, no lamenting the fate of the undead, no swooping, no capes, and no bats. Watching the film, one has to wonder how "vampire," as a reliable stand-in for a number of societal ills, becomes such a powerful metaphor, which can be deployed to signify themes as disparate as violent gangs or infectious diseases. Caleb's father, after he finds his son, administers a full blood transfusion in order to cure the infectious disease that led Caleb to a life of murder. It works, and Caleb becomes human once more, absolved of his former crimes. Later, the gang is destroyed except for Mae, who is also saved through blood transfusion. The movie ends with her and Caleb enjoying the sunrise—normalcy restored to the heartland. While in previous chapters I dealt with nonfiction representations of blood and pandemic, here I argue that films are powerful representations of cultural anxieties about diseases. *Near Dark* was one of many films released in the 1980s and 1990s that deployed vampires as allegories for HIV/AIDS pandemic. In this chapter, I argue that vampires serve as cultural metaphors for how society classifies and manages diseased and deviant bodies. Specifically, I use *Interview with the Vampire: The Vampire Chronicles* (Geffen & Jordan, 1994), *Blade* (Arad, Calamari, Harris, Lee & Norrington, 1998), and *John Carpenter's Vampires* (Potter & Carpenter, 1998) as case studies for how vampire films mapped on cultural discourse of the HIV/AIDS pandemic.

Monsters and Disease

The word *monster* takes its root from the Latin *monstra* meaning to "show forth," "warn," or "sign." It shares its root with "demonstrate," and from the beginning, teratology, or the science of monsters, has been preoccupied with understanding exactly what monsters demonstrate about their creation. The determination of causes of monstrosity was always an exercise in control and management of bodies and identities.

For example, Marie-Hélène Huet, in her influential book *Monstrous Imagination* (1993), writes of a persistent line of thought that argued that monstrous children were the result of maternal imagination. Instead of reflecting the father's image, as nature intended, monstrous children were the result of violent desires affecting the mother at the time of conception and throughout pregnancy. For example, according to Huet, Aristotle argued that a female was already a deviation from the norm, albeit a necessary one. The monster, however, was a gratuitous and useless variation on the norm. Aristotle presents "a definition of monstrosity that was primarily linked not to physical imperfections but rather to a deficiency in the natural and visible link between genitors and their progeny.... Though the monster was first defined as that which did not resemble him who engendered it, it nevertheless displayed some sort of resemblance, albeit a *false* resemblance, to an object external to its conception.... The maternal imagination erased the legitimate father's image from his offspring and thus created a monster" (Huet, 1993, pp. 4, 8). In a "normal" conception, semen played an active role, inputting generational material into a fertile and nurturing womb. Monstrous birth was then the result of a woman, through the power of her imagination, contributing to the generational process. Monstrous births were a mechanism of control and maintenance of appropriate gender roles.

In the sixteenth century, teratology became a province of classificatory medical sciences. The text which first classified monstrosity according to then-scientific guidelines, was Ambroise Paré's *De Monstres et prodiges* (*On Monsters and Marvels*, 1840). In it, Paré implemented a scientific medical approach to classify monstrous bodies according to three major categories: anomalies of excess (extra body parts), default (lack of body parts), and duplicity (Siamese twins) (Davidson, 1991; Huet, 1993; Leroi, 2003; Shildrick, 2002). Paré listed thirteen causes of monsters:

> The first is the glory of God. The second, his wrath. The third, too great a quantity of semen. The fourth, too small a quantity. The fifth, imagination. The sixth, the narrowness of the womb. The seventh, the unbecoming sitting position of the mother, who, while pregnant, remains seated too long with her thighs crossed or pressed against her stomach. The eighth, by a fall or blows struck against the stomach of the mother during pregnancy. The ninth, by hereditary or accidental illnesses. The tenth, by the rotting or corruption of the semen. The eleventh, by the mingling or mixture of seed. The twelfth, by the artifice or wandering beggars. The thirteenth, by demons or devils. (1982, pp. 3–4)

Davidson (1991) observes that the language of horror is absent from his descriptions, and Leroi (2003) points out that "*Des monstres* marks the presence of a new idea: that the causes of deformity must be sought in nature" (p. 7). Asma (2009) argues that Paré's classification points toward a more naturalistic explanation of monsters and that the next century marked a transition in the mechanization of nature where "the human body, now conceptualized as an elegant machine, became increasingly anatomized, analyzed, and understood. And the pathologies of that body, the monsters, became an important means by which the new surgeons and physicians could limn the *normal* laws of nature" (p. 149). While the timing of this transition is arguable, it is true that monsters started to increasingly serve as illustrations of the fallibility of nature—diseases, viruses, and pandemics, as opposed to the will of God or other supernatural forces. For example, vampires became integrated into the community narrative by losing many supernatural traits, such as an ability to transform him/herself into a bat or a wolf, virtually absent in contemporary vampire stories. Vampires still possess superhuman powers, but they are not as easily distinguishable from humans as they once were. Zanger (1997) argues that that a contemporary vampire is not the metaphysical evil of Bram Stoker, but rather the social deviant of Anne Rice. The new vampire has become socialized, humanized, and secularized. This transforms vampires from a site of cosmic conflict between God and Satan into an expression of individual personality, thus allowing for the existence of "safe" and "unsafe" vampires (Campbell, 2013). Much like model citizens, safe vampires are recognized for their work against their inherit wickedness and for the good of the human community. They use their powers in often-vain hopes to earn a right of belonging. These fictional explorations of differences between good and evil vampires have mapped well onto discourses of the HIV/AIDS pandemic.

Vampires, Disease, and HIV/AIDS

The myth of the vampire, or the dead coming back to feed on the living, had initially found its strongest expression in Eastern Europe, where nearly identical accounts about these creatures appeared from the sixteenth through the eighteenth century (Riccardo, 1994). There is also evidence of the vampiric legend in other parts of the world, such as the *langsuyar* in Malaysia, the *lamiai* in Greece, and the *chiang-shih* in China (Melton, 1994). There is a common element to these stories—a connection between vampires, disease, and deviance. Melton (1994) writes, "[T]he vampire figure in folklore emerged as an answer to otherwise unsolvable problems within culture. The vampire was seen as the cause of certain unexplainable evils, accounted for the appearance of some extraordinary occurrences within the society, and was often cited as the end product of some extraordinary behavior" (p. 445). The *langsuyar* and the *lamiai* were women who gave birth to a stillborn child and become vampires out of grief. Children with birth defects were also considered candidates for vampirehood. Vampires were also a part of grieving process—the dead, if not properly buried, were believed to come back to life to deal with unfinished family business (Melton, 1994). In all of these instances, vampires served as a mechanism for social control. Thus, "People who stepped outside of the moral and religious boundaries of the community not only jeopardized their souls, but could have become vampires" (Melton, 1994, p. 446). The vampire stories are nearly universal in the global communication. As I discussed in chapter two, the media in Nicaragua used the trope of the vampire to communicate its outrage over shady blood-bank practices. Vampire narratives also appear in the oral histories collected by the anthropologists Luise White (1993) in Uganda, which told of white people who captured Africans and extracted their blood. The stories' use of vampire myths and metaphors suggested that between 1918 and 1925, vampires appeared in Uganda and used needles to suck the blood of Africans; the vampires sold or drank the blood while their victims died. Although these stories were embedded in the colonial context of power and exploitation, White argues against reducing them to simple parables of the "oppressor" and the "oppressed." Looking instead at the vampire as an epistemological category with which Africans described their world, he argues that "these vampires are not simply generalized metaphors of extraction and oppression but that these images are, like other orally transmitted information, told at specific times to specific people for specific reasons" (White, 1993, p. 29). These are but two examples of global vampire narratives. Nelkin (1999) writes, "Variations in the vampire myth have appeared in many other contexts where there are social tensions, for they serve as a way to identity the sources of danger and to place blame. They appeared, for example in the nineteenth-century blood libel stories about Jews who purportedly killed Christian boys and used their blood to make matzoh during the Passover holidays" (p. 283).

The vampire was seen as a diseased and deviant member of a community who was guilty of violating norms and values. In fact, vampires have always served as metaphors of disease and infection. Gordon, Hollinger, and Aldiss (1997) write that, in the nineteenth century, vampires were analogies of symptoms of tuberculosis: "Consider its associations with wasting, with paleness, with the flow of blood from the mouth, night restlessness, alternate burning and chills, even with the victim's rumored sexual activity" (p. 6). Melton (1994) notes that tuberculosis was a deadly disease with no known cause or cure, which, as a result, became a subject of occult speculations. Vampires were seen as an explanation for this affliction. Even Bram Stoker's *Dracula* (1997) can be read as a cautionary tale of blood disease. Dika (1996) writes, "The notion of a blood disease and of the plague, however, has been, from the beginning, associated with Dracula. In Stoker's novel, Dracula is a polluting force, spreading death and defilement through the blood (Mina even says, 'There is a poison in my blood, in my soul, which may destroy me'), and in *Nosferatu*, the Count is specifically credited with the spread of the Black Death" (Dika, 1996, p. 394). However, the most compelling element of vampire-related disease is a conflation of infection and sex.

Vampires' feeding has historically been viewed as a sexual act, which, in recent decades, increasingly has been seen as homoerotic (Schopp, 1997). For example, Taubin (1995) analyzes *Interview with the Vampire: The Vampire Chronicles* (Geffen & Jordan, 1994) as "the story of an exceedingly longtime companionship, of a marriage between two men which begins in the heat of passion (when Lestat first sinks his teeth into Louis' neck, they fly heavenward locked in each other's arms) and which then settles into a daily routine of naggings, recriminations, and betrayals without ever losing its symbiotic pull" (p. 11). The act of siring, or creating other vampires, takes place outside of the usual male/female matrix. Vampire relationships subvert heteronormative ideals of family and birth. They show alternative ways of organizing one's life. Wood (1996) argues that Dracula is such a potent cultural symbol because of an exhibition of "perverse" sexualities, such as promiscuity and bisexuality. Dresser (1989) claims that the fans respond the most to vampires' sexual otherness. He writes, "The vampire's sexual otherness both reflects and fosters a desire to break free from sexual constraints....The vampire appeals to fans because it transgresses boundaries and challenges the constraints that we face every day" (as cited in Schopp, 1997, p. 233).

While vampires serve as metaphors for "perverse" sexuality, their monstrosity (and their power), first and foremost, is tied to blood. In fact, vampires' sexuality is drenched in blood and the desire for blood turns vampires into monsters. Freeland (2000) makes explicit a connection between blood and vampire sexuality, explaining that "vampires are polymorphously perverse: In their search for blood, they can find physical intimacy with a person of almost any gender, age, race, or social class. Sexuality is transmuted into a new kind of exchange of bodily fluids where reproduction, if it occurs at all, confers the 'dark gift' of immortal undead existence rather than natural birth" (p. 124), and Carol Corbin and Robert Campbell (1999) write that in the film *Bram Stoker's Dracula* (Apted, O'Connor & Coppola 1992), "Sex is blood, blood is lineage, and lineage is romantic love" (p. 43).

Popular vampire narratives should be analyzed, therefore, as policing devices, which illustrate how those with tainted blood and perverse desires affect a community. What makes vampires a particularly powerful metaphor is precisely their ability to represent different identities, bodies, and social problems. In popular culture, vampires are stand-ins for viruses, infectious diseases, perverse sexualities, tainted blood, impure racial and ethnic identities, and other so-called deviances. Judith Halberstam (1995), for example, writes about the economy of gothic sexuality and vampire identity:

> Blood circulates throughout vampiric sexuality as a substitute or metaphor for other bodily fluids (milk, semen) and once again, the leap between bad blood and perverse sexuality is not hard to make....Gothic sexuality, furthermore, manifests itself as a kind of technology, a productive force which transforms the blood of the native into the lust of the other, and as an economy which unites the threat of the foreign and perverse within a single, monstrous body. (p. 101)

Halberstam argues that Gothic monsters, such as Dracula, unite fears about race, sexuality, and the perverse into a single body. The reason why Dracula exhibits all the stereotypes of the nineteenth-century Jew, Halberstam contends, is precisely because in the figure of a Jew, "Gothic fiction finds a monster versatile enough to represent fears about race, nation, and sexuality, a monster who combines in one body fears of the foreign and the perverse" (p. 14). It is therefore the cultural construction of blood as a determinant of national identity that gave rise to Stoker's account of Dracula. Dracula is a foreigner who embodies fears of blood contamination, foreign identity, and perverse sexuality. Indeed, as Halberstam argues, with the rise of bourgeois society, the blood of nobility was reconstructed as the blood of the native and both were identified in contradiction to "impure" races. Historical battles over the purity of national identity allowed for staging battles within a body. In her analysis, Sue-Ellen Case (2000) argues that at that time, life itself "was formulated through a legal, literary, and scientific discourse on blood, which stabilized privilege by affirming the right to life for those who could claim blood and further, pure blood, and the consequent death sentence, either metaphorically or literally, for those who could not" (p. 200).

Dracula embodied dangers of hybridity and an anxiety over reverse colonization, an invasion by primitive force (Arata, 1990). Halberstam writes, "Gothic anti-Semitism makes the Jew a monster with bad blood and it defines monstrosity as a mixture of bad blood, unstable gender identity, sexual and economic parasitism, and degeneracy" (p. 89). In *Dracula*, vampires are the race that weakens the English heritage through sexual degeneracy and the disease of blood lust. And much like the blood discourses in which they are steeped, vampire narratives manage difference, or in this case, monstrosity, through politics of exclusion, elimination, or incorporation. Much like in *Near Dark* (Feldman, Nabatoff & Bigelow, 1987), at the end of *Dracula*, Dracula is destroyed and Mina is incorporated back into a heteronormative British society. However, a connection between blood, sexuality, and vampires has found new life in popular narratives of AIDS. Much like vampires themselves, HIV/AIDS is a pandemic of signification, combining a deadly and mysterious disease with the dangers of bad blood and perverse sexual practices.

I argued in the previous chapter that the early association between HIV/AIDS and male homosexuality irrevocably shaped society's response to the disease. Even as AIDS moved into the so-called "general" population, it was viewed, and continues to be seen, as affecting those on the margins. Stories of AIDS told of an attack by an alien—and monstrous—virus, and by those dangerous Others who engaged in perverse sexual practices. These terrors rivaled those of a good horror film and together they mapped onto a cinematic portrayal of a vampire. After all, this was a creature whose desires were considered to be perverse and whose body was historically connected to disease and death. They were mysterious creatures of the night who could seduce humans, bring them to ecstasy, and leave them dead or diseased. Chaudhuri (1997) writes:

> This exposition of an alien [vampiric] entity transmitted by the blood, inducing progressive mutation—internally colonizing the body's cells, which then work against the good of the body—cannot escape comparison with AIDS. It matches the 'scientific' version of how HIV transforms the cells of the body: docking with the T-cell, it transcribes its genetic information onto the host cell's own genetic code, so that each time a host cell divides, viral copies are produced along with more host cells each containing the viral code. The virus and vampirism substitute themselves for the essence, so that the immune system confronted by the onslaught of simulacra, is disarmed and can no longer recognize the enemies within; this engenders a terrifying epistemological ambiguity, for the immune system, dedicated to telling the difference between Self and Non-Self, can no longer make these distinctions. (p. 189)

The homoerotic element of vampire fiction and cinema made the association between vampirism and HIV/AIDS easy to draw. For example, Nixon (1997) argues that the vampire movie *The Hunger* (1983), released about two years into the AIDS epidemic, is a stunning allegory of the disease in its portrayal of sexual desire and infection. She writes:

> There is something eerily familiar about the scenario of a seemingly-beautiful, charmingly-anonymous lover who, during an unusually passionate sexual encounter, transmits some virulent infection that cannot even be diagnosed, let alone cured.... New York nightclubs and leather bars, anonymous sex with invisibly-infected strangers, transmitted and undiagnosable blood diseases that transform cells and have some sort of connection to lethal viruses afflicting monkeys, and same-sex sexuality add up, now, to only one thing. (p. 117)

Much like journalistic and documentary narratives of the HIV/AIDS pandemic, vampire films serve as a mechanism of social, political, and cultural control. Vampire films create a seamless narrative of community in which difference is managed through exclusion and incorporation. In these films, vampires have to struggle against their identity and sexual desires. Moreover, as scientific knowledge of the HIV/AIDS pandemic has evolved, so did the cure for vampirism. *Near Dark* (Feldman, Nabatoff & Bigelow, 1987) cured vampirism with blood transfusions and *Blade* (Arad et al., 1998) used a serum, not unlike AZTs. In other words, as cultural and scientific discourses of AIDS changed, so did vampire films. In the rest of the chapter, I trace these changes through the analysis of *Interview with the Vampire: The Vampire Chronicles* (Geffen & Jordan, 1994), *Blade* (Arad et al., 1998), and *John Carpenter's Vampires* (Potter & Carpenter, 1998), illustrating how vampire cinema represented societal attitudes about HIV/AIDS.

Interview with the Vampire (1994)

Interview with the Vampire, based on Anne Rice's book of the same name, is structured as a flashback told to a reporter by a two-century-old vampire Louis (Brad Pitt). The story begins in 1791 Louisiana where Louis, grieving over the death of his wife and daughter, meets Lestat (Tom Cruise), a vampire who offers him an eternal life, free of grief and pain. Louis accepts Lestat's offer, but forever regrets his choice and cannot bring himself to kill humans, feeding instead on the blood of rats and pigeons. Finally, overcome by his urges, he drinks from a young girl named Claudia. Louis leaves the girl for dead, but Lestat makes her into a vampire, creating, in his words, "one big happy family." As decades pass, Claudia, enraged at being trapped in a child's body, develops a close relationship with Louis, and becomes resentful of Lestat, finally attempting to kill him.

Scholars have read *Interview with the Vampire* as a story of a gay relationship. For example, Taubin (1995) provided the following summary of the movie:

> *Interview with the Vampire* is the story of an exceedingly longtime companionship, of a marriage between two men which begins in the heat of passion (when Lestat first sinks his teeth into Louis' neck, they fly heavenward locked in each other's arms) and which then settles into a daily routine of naggings, recriminations and betrayals without ever losing its symbiotic pull. (p. 11)

The film explicitly engages with homoerotic undertones. For example, Lestat is said to prefer young male victims, and when Louis meets Armand (Antonio Banderas), the world's oldest vampire, they all but profess their love for one another. Vampires also engage in other kinds of sexual activity. There are hints of incest: for example, Lestat creates Claudia by essentially making love to her. Claudia often refers to Louis as "my father, my lover," and when he finally consents to creating her a mother figure—an illusion of a normalized existence—she thanks him with a kiss, which comes across not as a daughter's gratitude, but rather as a sexual rite of passage. There are other hints of "inappropriate" desire: Armand's boy-servant's arms are covered with "love" bites.

Louis is the only fully sympathetic character in the film, precisely because he is haunted by angst and guilt over what he has become: "a killer" who "belongs in hell." Consumed by self-hatred, he looks for meaning and fails to find it. Wanting, yet unable, to fight his thirst, he laments, "Am I damned? Am I from the devil? Is my very nature that of a devil? And all the while, as these dreaded questions caused me to neglect my thirst, my thirst grew hotter, my veins were threads of pain in my flesh, my temples throbbed." He is disgusted by his own "perverse" desires, but he cannot fight them. His own blood overcomes him. Whereas Lestat embraces his monstrosity, Louis is repulsed by it. He cannot find peace in what he has become, and he does not want to inflict his existence on anyone else. Louis's interview, the basis for the film's story, is Louis's attempt to justify his existence and desires to the human world. The audience is expected to sympathize and pity Louis because he cannot help being a vampire *and* because he hates himself. Louis can become integrated into a human community only as a cautionary tale; his redemption lies in self-hatred.

The metaphor of vampirism as an infectious disease is grounded in these allegories of "perverse" desires and self-loathing. In *Interview with the Vampire*, the vampire virus is contained within a community of perverse Others. Their victims, be they slaves, street people, or prostitutes, are located on the margins of society and therefore are inconsequential. Much like the American cultural discourse of AIDS was not able to shake divisions between "innocent" and "guilty" victims, or between those whose identities were implicated in the disease and those who were not, so does *Interview with the Vampire* make much of the choice to become a vampire, or drink vampire's blood, in order to be turned. Lestat insists on a verbal agreement with Louis; he tells him, "I will give you a choice I never had." Louis' choice is visually symbolized in his embrace of Lestat during their first encounter as they fly towards heavens in an orgasmic display of pleasure, danger, and desire. Wolf (1997) writes about victims' stillness in

Dracula films: "Stillness emphasizes the passivity of the victim, who therefore cannot be held responsible for being victimized....In no [*Dracula* movies] do we see a victim embracing the vampire at the moment that he or she takes blood" (pp. 255–256). Lestat himself was not given a choice to become a vampire and this is the reason why he is free of guilt about his "monstrosity"—he did not choose it. Herein lies Louis' damnation—he chose a risky behavior of vampirism which condemned him to be the infected Other for all eternity.

Interview with the Vampire argues, therefore, that the infected Others are condemned to lives of self-loathing as a result of their own choices and behavior. And while there are subversive possibilities in the vampires' desires and relationships, they are never fully realized. In fact, the film warns its audience, as personified by the reporter Malloy (Christian Slater), not to be seduced by vampire lifestyle. As Louis ends his story, Malloy begs to be a part of it:

MALLOY : No...it can't end like that...
LOUIS : But it has. There is no more to tell.
MALLOY : But you talk about passion, about longing, about things I'll never know in my life! It's still inside you, in every syllable you speak! And then you tell me it ends like that? Just empty?
LOUIS : It's over, I'm telling you...
MALLOY : You need a new passion, Louis, a new reason to feel...what a story you've told, you don't understand yourself.
LOUIS : Do what you want with it. Learn what you can. Give the story to others.
MALLOY : You have another chance, Louis. Take me! Give me your gift, your power...
LOUIS : Is this what you want? You ask me for this after all I've told you?
MALLOY : If I could see what you've seen, feel what you've felt I wouldn't let it end like this! You need a like to the world out there, a connection...then it won't end like this...You need me.
LOUIS : Dear God. I've failed again, haven't I?

Louis threatens Malloy with death as the punishment for failing to grasp his lesson and the audience is warned against the dangers of being seduced by sexual desires. At the end of the film, the virus is contained, and those infected are damned to suffer for the rest of the eternity.

Blade (1998)

In *Interview with the Vampire*, the vampiric virus is contained amongst risk groups, but in *Blade* (Arad et al., 1998), the infection has spread. *Blade* represents a change in scientific and cultural understanding of HIV/AIDS and those affected. Blade (Wesley Snipes) is an African American vampire slayer. He is a hybrid: half human and half vampire. A vampire bit Blade's mother while she was pregnant. She died, but not before Blade was born with "all of vampires' strengths and none of the weaknesses." Blade can exist in the sunlight, but he still craves blood. As a homeless child, he fed on humans before Whistler (Kris Kristofferson)—a man whose family was killed by vampires—took him in and brought him up to be a vampire slayer. We are introduced to vampire culture early on in the film. A female vampire leads her unsuspecting male victim to an S&M leather club located in the basement of a meatpacking factory. Young, attractive people of various sexual orientations rave the night away. As the music grows louder, the sprinkler system is activated, but instead of water, it showers dancers with blood. This scene sets up the rest of the film: *Blade* is practically steeped in blood, disease, and race.

In the film, vampirism is represented as an acquired blood virus. As hematologist Karen Jenson (N'Bushe Wright) analyzes a charred body, she looks at blood through the microscope and immediately identifies it as "not human blood." She proceeds to explain, "The red blood cells are biconvex, which is theoretically impossible. They're hypochromic, there's virtually no hemoglobin in them. Look at the PMNs, they're binucleated; they should be mononucleated." This is an example of what John Jordan (1999) calls "the scientization of the vampire mystique" (p. 11). Throughout the film, the vampire virus is articulated and legitimized through scientific discourse. The audience is supposed to suspend disbelief in vampires because of scientific proof offered for their existence. Even vampire weaknesses are defined in scientific terms: crosses—the symbol of the old, religious mystique—do nothing, but vampires are "severely allergic" to the UV-ray component of sunlight.

Moreover, vampirism is analogous to the HIV/AIDS virus. Karen spews in the face of Deacon Frost (played by Stephen Dorff), Blade's arch vampire nemesis: "You are a virus, an STD." Blade has to take a serum to fight the vampire virus in his own blood—a remarkable parallel to AZTs or protease inhibitors. This is a painful process, as his vampire infection is hard to beat. Whistler explains Blade's condition to Karen:

WHISTLER : Blade's unique, you know. A one in a billion anomaly. He can withstand sunlight, garlic, even silver. But he still has the thirst.

KAREN : What happens if he doesn't take the serum?

WHISTLER : The thirst overcomes him, just like the others. It's not something he can control. The problem is, time's running out. His body's starting to reject the serum. And so far, all my efforts to find a cure have ended in failure—

Here the virus can overtake a person and cause the thirst, which, results in infection and the death of others. Anyone could be bitten and therefore infected. The virus, coupled with the desire, the thirst, associated with the virus, develops an identity of its own; it *becomes* the infected person. Much like in *Interview with the Vampire*, *Blade* portrays desire as dangerous and ultimately deadly. The virus turns a person into a monster and he or she becomes immediately responsible for his or her monstrosity. Interestingly enough, *Blade* distinguishes between those infected with the vampire virus and those born with it. Here the film plays with eugenics and the concept of pure blood. The film introduces the vampire governing council, the House of Erabus. The head of the council, a thin white man with piercing blue eyes named Dragonetti, speaks with a European (and slightly German) accent. Members of the council are born vampires and, therefore, are considered to be pure bloods. At the end of the movie, Deacon Frost kills Dragonetti and releases the Blood God who threatens to turn everyone into a vampire, thus erasing the line between pure and turned vampires.

Blade's fear of the virus is thus based in paranoia. Vampires are said to have made a deal with the government and therefore are allowed to function as normal or human members of society. Blade explains to Karen, "There is a real world behind this one and if you want to survive it, you better learn to pull a trigger.... They [vampires] have their claws in everything: politics, finance, and real estate. They already own half of the downtown." Vampires also apparently own blood banks in every major city. This paranoia runs parallel to the anti-Semitic discourse associated with *Dracula*. However, it also indicates a fear of otherness run rampant throughout society. Unlike *Interview with the Vampire*, in *Blade*, disease is not contained in a few "perverse" Others. Because of government's inaction and enabling, the virus spreads to the streets, corporations, and blood banks. After Karen is exposed to the truth about the vampires, she wanders the streets, staring suspiciously at people, looking for any hint that they might too be infected. In *Blade* the virus has spread to the general population and there is only one person, Blade, who can identify the infected on sight. This is because he is one of them.

Much like Louis in *Interview with the Vampire*, Blade is enveloped in self-loathing. He says, "I am not human, humans do not drink blood. I have spent my whole life looking for that thing that killed my mother. It made me what I am and every time I take one of these monsters out, I get a piece of my life back." Blade is represented as a tragic figure destroyed by his otherness. He has to constantly undergo a painful medical procedure in order to fight the spread of virus inside the body. He is sympathetic because, much like Louis, he has recognized and chosen to fight the evil which lurks within him. In the film, Blade is left with two choices: he can either fight the virus with medication and the love of a good woman, or to embrace his otherness and join the vampires. Deacon Frost invites Blade to join him:

FROST : Why not? The future of our race runs through your bloodstream. You've got the best of both worlds, Blade. All of our strengths and none of our weaknesses.

BLADE : Maybe I don't see it that way.

FROST : Oh, so it's back to pretending we're human again, is it? Spare me the Uncle Tom routine. You can't keep denying what you are. You're one of us, Blade. You always have been.

BLADE : You're wrong.

FROST : Am I? You think the humans will ever accept a half-breed like you? They can't. They're afraid of you. (*pointedly*) The humans fear us because we're superior. They fear us because in their hearts they know their race has become obsolete.

Frost's reference to "the Uncle Tom routine" draws a parallel between being an African American in a predominantly white society and being a half-vampire in a predominantly human world. As an African American vampire hunter, Blade is doomed to live on the margins of the society.

Interview with the Vampire was set exclusively in the vampire world, which sexualized their "perverse" desire, making vampirism appealing to human outsiders such as Malloy. This is not the case in *Blade*, and while most of its main vampire characters are very attractive, the vampire bite itself loses its sensuality and is instead shown as a grizzly, murderous act. The only time in the film when the vampire bite is portrayed as a sexual act is when Karen makes Blade bite her in order to restore his strength. Here, the desire and blood lust is legitimized through its association with heterosexuality. It is a heterosexual sex act, which restores Blade's strength and, in turn, saves the world from the spread of the virus. It also renews Blade's sense of purpose to fight vampires and his own vampire identity. The analogies to the AIDS pandemic are plentiful in the film: the inability to detect those who are infected, the lack of the cure, the ineffectiveness of medication, the anger towards government irresponsiveness, and the fear of blood banks. Moreover, vampires are portrayed as purely evil; they are directly implicated in their monstrosity and they relish infecting and killings others. The lesson of *Blade* is that when monsters are everywhere, we have no choice but to destroy them all.

John Carpenter's Vampires (1998)

John Carpenter's Vampires (Potter & Carpenter, 1998) further extends the analogies and metaphors of previous films in the genre. In *Interview with the Vampire* and *Blade*, vampires possessed distinct personalities, while in *Vampires* they are presented as an undifferentiated, evil mass whose bite, however minor, will automatically transform a person into a vampire. In this film vampires *are* the virus; they do not have an existence outside of the disease. Here, the deviant or perverse Other is merged with the disease; there is no distinction drawn between the two. The virus has gained a life of its own as a creature ready to strike and kill at will.

In *Vampires*, the pandemic is recast as a battle between diseased and healthy male bodies. James Woods plays Jack Crow, a vampire hunter for hire, who leads a crew of vampire-slaying roughnecks. The justification for Crow's occupation is pure revenge. After vampires killed his parents, the Catholic church raised him to be a vampire hunter. Much like Blade, Jack Crow is portrayed as a quintessential heterosexual male, down to a laconic speech pattern punctuated by grunts. There are extensive shots of Jack Crow's bulging crotch as he strolls into various vampire layers and kills their inhabitants. His macho gang also enjoys vampire slaying. One of the running jokes in the film is that killing a vampire gives one "wood." The killing of the diseased Other is portrayed as a masculine act where healthy heterosexual masculinity is contrasted to vampire sexual deviance. There are no female characters of consequences in the film since there is no place for a woman in the battle of masculinities.

The film references previous vampire representations to illustrate its own vampire *vérité*. Jack Crow explains to a new recruit, "They [the vampires] are not romantic. It is not like they are a bunch of fucking fags hopping around in rented formalwear and seducing everyone in sight with cheesy Eurotrash accent. Forget everything you have seen in the movies." This reference to films like *Interview with the Vampire* establishes *Vampires* as a grim, and homophobic, reality. There is no room for sympathy or understanding; the boundary between normal and deviant desires must be solidified at all costs. *Vampires* deepens *Blade*'s determination to destroy all vampires. Whereas Blade still discusses what it means to be a vampire, Jack Crow simply destroys. There is also an exaggerated paranoia directed towards the authority, in this case the Catholic Church, which has encouraged the virus to grow. In *Vampires*, however, there are no liminal or ambiguous vampire figures, like Louis or Blade. The virus must be destroyed, and so must any of its carriers. It cannot be contained or assimilated, and vampires must die in the effort to keep the human community healthy.

The changes in these films reflect the evolution of the HIV/AIDS pandemic and the shift in the associated popular, scientific, and cultural discourses. *Interview with the Vampire* portrays the vampire as mostly contained within a small community of deviant "Others," whose infections are a direct consequence of their perverse desires. *Blade* reflects cultural paranoia over the spread of the disease into the general population. With the help, or at least the negligent inaction, of government, vampires have assimilated into society and become undistinguishable from humans. *John Carpenter's Vampires* builds on *Blade's* paranoia and casts the battle against the disease into the terms of "healthy" versus "diseased" bodies. The vampires have lost all identity separate from the virus; they become the virus. In all of these films, however, vampires are implicated in their own monstrosity. They are responsible for either giving in to or resisting their sexualized urges, and their identities are inseparable from their infected blood. These portrayals carry consequences, for they can provide us with an understanding of how "deviant" or "abnormal" bodies are managed through mediated discourse, and, as these films illustrate, the choices are few. The "Others" can either be kept on the margins (*Interview with the Vampire)*; assimilated, as long as they use their powers for our good (*Blade)*; or destroyed (*Vampires*). These popular representations go hand in hand with the mechanisms of cultural exclusion/incorporation discussed in previous chapters. Steeped in blood metaphors and viral discourses, these mechanisms and their representations are used to classify, control, and manage the bodies and identities of those who do not belong.

Michel Foucault (1980) writes that, at certain historical, moments, one can observe the emergence of a new regime of knowledge. We must then ask, "How is it that at certain moments and in certain orders of knowledge there are these sudden take-offs, these hastenings of evolution, these transformations which fail to correspond to the calm, continuist image that is normally accredited?" It's a matter of knowing "what effects of power circulate among scientific statements, what constitutes, as it were, their internal regime of power, and how and why at certain moments that regime undergoes a global modification" (pp. 112–113). The call to understand mechanisms through which new regimes of knowledge come to be is strikingly similar to Judith Halberstam's (1995) examination of the mechanisms through which the vampire came to embody the production of sexuality. She writes, "The vampire represents the productions of sexuality itself.... The point really is not to figure out which so-called perverse sexuality Dracula or the vampire in general embodies, rather we should identify the mechanism by which the consuming monster who reproduces his own image comes to represent the construction of sexuality itself" (p. 100). In other words, in order to understand how disease functions in society, we must direct our attention to the society's mediated construction and representation of its monsters. As Nina Auerbach argues, every age gets the vampire it deserves (1997).

· 4 ·

GLOBALIZATION, PANDEMICS, AND THE PROBLEM OF SECURITY

The film *Contagion* (King, Polaire, Skoll & Soderbergh, 2011) opens with a cough and ends with a handshake. In between, it is a story of the world struggling to keep itself infection-free in the age of globalization, and a story of security and governance in the time of pandemic. In this chapter, I explore media representations of pandemic as a social and cultural site where the problems of governance, security, and risk are presented and resolved. Starting with *Contagion* and proceeding into fictional and nonfictional accounts of avian flu and SARS, I argue that, as a global crisis, pandemics demonstrate the anticipatory nature of risk and the immediate biopolitical problem of governance. Media narratives, therefore, attempt to reconcile the present danger with the future risk. They make the present future-perfect.

Contagion and the Biosecurity of the Population

When *Contagion* was released in 2011, it was a subject of reviews, not only in the usual entertainment and film magazines, but also in numerous scientific and public health journals. Since the filmmakers laid claim to a relative veracity, these reviews wanted to know if the portrayals were accurate and if the science was good. Overall, the reviewers were satisfied with both. Shah (2011) of *Lancet* proclaims "Public health education has never had it so good.... *Contagion* is deliciously authentic." Mueller (2011) of *Science* writes, "*Contagion* is familiar terrain for Hollywood, but the interesting twist here is that this time Hollywood decided to let scientists in on the script. The result is a gripping yet refreshingly accurate warning about the very real threat of zoonotic disease and the potential impact a rapidly emerging pandemic could have on society." The accuracy of representations was widely attributed to Ian Lipkin of Columbia University, an expert in emerging infectious disease and the co-chair of CDC's National Biosurveillance Advisory Subcommitee, who served as an advisor to the script. In an interview with Krisberg (2011) of *The Nation's Health*, a publication of the American Public Health Association, Lipkin tells readers that "the science is really very good. We took sequences of known viruses and we modeled them and morphed them into this new virus, but everything you see is biologically plausible." And Scott Burns, the film's screenwriter, said about the process of making a film about a pandemic and public health, "I became acutely aware of how there is a shared health of a society" (Krisberg, 2011).

The securing of that shared health is what I refer to here as the biosecurity of the population, or what Lakoff and Collier (2008) call the various political and technological interventions and efforts to "secure health." *Contagion* portrays the zoonotic—transmitted from animals to humans—virus as a threat to the shared health of the global community. The threat is a direct result of globalization, both in the origin of the disease and in its mode of transmission. The origin of the disease is attributed to an instance where "somewhere in the world, the wrong pig met up with the wrong bat," and this statement by a CDC scientist is revealed to be true at the end of the film, which portrays how the clearing of a native forest near Hong Kong disrupts the bat population. Bats scatter, and one of them flies into a nearby pigpen, where one of the pigs subsequently eats a banana brought in by the bat. The pig is then taken to slaughter and handled by a chef who does not wash his hands. The chef then shakes hands with Beth Emhoff (Gwyneth Paltrow), our patient zero from Minneapolis, Minnesota, who carries the disease into the Western world. During her layover in Chicago, where she has sex with an ex-boyfriend, Beth touches bar snacks, and a bartender takes her credit card. The camera lingers on these details to show how ordinary contact can easily endanger shared health. Suddenly, the scene changes to Kowloon, Hong Kong (population 2.1 million, according to the caption), then to London, England (population 8.6 million), then to Tokyo, Japan (population 33.6 million), and finally rests in Minneapolis, Minnesota (population 3.3 million), where Beth gets home to her husband

and hugs her son. In each locale, there is a clearly ill person who has been infected through an interaction with Beth and who is now endangering the health of the number of people projected on the screen. As I illustrate later in the chapter's discussion of SARS, it is not arbitrary that Hong Kong is the point of origin for the film's pandemic. It was picked specifically because of its status as a global city, as well as the presupposed exoticism of the types of animals being slaughtered, as well as the perceived conditions of slaughtering. We see similar characterizations in Beth's marital infidelity—a seemingly unnecessary plot point; in the global reach of the virus; in the attribution of its spread to the uncivilized practices of the East; in the tale of heroic Western scientists battling the virus despite obstruction efforts of their respective governments; and, of course, in the tale's Chinese militia, who take an epidemiologist hostage to make sure that their village receives the vaccine. These are all a part of what Wald (2008) describes as imagined communities formed by disease. She writes, "While the experts are busy tracking the microbes, the disease does its own work of revelation, making visible the social interactions of the imagined community. Microbes tell the often hidden story of who has been where and when, and of what they did there. *Contagion*, that is, charts social interactions that are often not otherwise visible" (p. 35). Here, she draws on the work of Benedict Anderson (2006), who, in the influential book *Imagined Communities*, argues that nation-ness is a cultural artifact and that the nation needs to be understood as an imagined political community. It is imaginary because "in the minds of each [member of the nation] lives the image of their communion," and it is imagined as a community because regardless of inequality or exploitation, "the nation is always conceived as a deep, horizontal comradeship" (pp. 6, 7). Most importantly for our purposes, Anderson argues that the cultural artifact of nation-ness, once created, becomes modular, "capable of being transplanted, with varying degrees of self-consciousness, to a great variety of social terrains to merge and be merged with a correspondingly wise variety of political and ideological constellations" (p. 4). If we apply the concept of imagined communities to the global world, then, together with mediated narratives of contagion, they illustrate how globality is constructed, insofar as whose bodies matter, whose identities are compromised, and how a population is rendered secure.

Another way the global imaginary and the problem of contagion can be conceptualized is through what Michel Foucault (2007), in his lectures on *Security, Territory, Population*, calls the milieu, or the problem of circulation and causality, which he contrasts with the discipline, or the problem of confinement and performance. He argues that the problem of a disease has become the problem of movement, where "the milieu appears as field of intervention in which…one tries to affect, precisely, a population…a multiplicity of individuals who are and fundamentally and essentially only exist biologically bound to the materiality within which they live" (p. 21). What we try to regulate through the milieu is "precisely the conjunction of a series of events produced by these individuals, populations, and groups, and quasi natural events which occur around them" (p. 21). The problem of the milieu is the problem of movement, or proper accounting for circumstances, causalities, and circulations, which form contagion as a medical and narrative problem. Mueller (2011) remarked that director Steven Soderbergh's technique of weaving together stories of individuals and organizations, while constantly moving across locales, worked well for the film because "it helps to build suspense as the film makes clear that the race to develop and implement a vaccine cannot match the pace at which society is crumbling. Viewers witness both the impact a highly transmissible pandemic virus that kills many of its victims has on the day-to-day lives of those affected and the broader effects it has on society. The director's approach also works because it shows how a pandemic could play out in today's world. What we see is not reassuring." The temporal and spatial jumps exemplify the problem of security and governance. The camera constantly focuses on the minute moments of the everyday life: a cup of coffee ordered, a table wiped, a document left on the table. As Mueller (2011) argues, "[B]y letting the camera linger just a little too long on a bus rail or a cup of coffee in a café, Soderbergh helps viewers appreciate how fast a virus such as this can spread." Dr. Erin Mears (Kate Winslet), an Epidemic Intelligence Service officer, tells officials in Minneapolis, as well as the audience, that the circulations and movements in the milieu are indeed the problem. She explains the concept of fomites as a transmission from surfaces: "The average person touches their face two or three thousand times a day. Three to five times every waking minute. In between, we're touching doorknobs, water fountains, elevator buttons, and each other. Those things become fomites."

The problem of securing the viral transmission, given the circulations of movements, gestures, and microbes, exemplifies the problem of security and governance. Foucault (2003) discusses this as the scientific, political, and biological problem of population, a problem aimed at the right to make live and let die, or a new technology of power—biopolitics of the human race. Biopolitics appeals to "man-as-species"; it governs on the level of life itself. The processes of life, such as the birth rate and the mortality rate, become political and economic problems, which are "biopolitics' first objects of knowledge and the targets it seeks to control" (p. 243). This problem of make live and let die plagues *Contagion* as the scientists attempt to quantify and control the mortality rate of the outbreak. Early on in the film, Dr. Mears is faced with the biopolitical problem of knowledge and regulation. As the government officials in Minneapolis are worried about an unnecessary panic and the economic fallout of announcing a possible pandemic, Mears is worried about accurately predicting the spread of infection in the population.

STATE OFFICIAL: We need to walk the governor through this before we freak everybody out. I mean, we can't even tell people right now what they should be afraid of.... It's the biggest shopping weekend of the year. And who stays home with the kids? People that work in stores? Government workers? People that work at hospitals? When will we know what this is? What causes it, what cures it? Things that keep people calm.

MEARS: What we need to determine is this: For every person who gets sick, how many other people are they likely to infect? So, for seasonal flu, that's usually about one. Smallpox, on the other hand, that's over three. Now, before we had a vaccine, polio spread at a rate between four and six. Now, we call that number the R-nought. R stands for the reproductive rate of the virus. How fast it multiplies depends on a variety of factors—the incubation period, how long a person is contagious. Sometimes people can be contagious without even having symptoms. We need to know that too. And we need to know how big the population of people susceptible to the virus might be.

The political, social, and economic problem of the population is the problem of securitization of the milieu. As Foucault (2003) writes, biopolitics' last domain is the control of human species as living being and "their environment, the milieu in which they live" (p. 245). This is a technology that does not center on the body as disciplinary technologies do, but upon life: "A technology which brings together the series of random events that can occur in a living mass, a technology which tries to predict the probability of those events, or at least to compensate for their effects. This is a technology which aims to establish a sort of homeostasis, not by training individuals, but *by achieving an overall equilibrium that protects the security of the whole from internal dangers* [emphasis added]" (p. 249).

While *Contagion* reifies biopolitical modes of regulation and security through scientific language, it also does so through seemingly unconnected "human interest" stories. One of the most interesting of these is the story of Beth's extramarital affair in Chicago, specifically because it seemingly does not fit with the rest of the film. She still could have been an index patient, her son could have still become infected and died, and her husband Mitch (Matt Damon) could have still had viral immunity and remained able to safeguard his daughter against the pandemic and societal breakdown which followed. The affair did not need to exist for the movie to make sense. So why was it included? I argue that this plot point illustrates media narratives' positioning within the global biopolitical system of regulation and security. There is an obvious moral to the story—Beth transgressed and she was punished. She was punished for being unfaithful, but also for being a working mom who enjoyed work trips and for being the breadwinner in the relationship (it is stated that Mitch is looking for a job, but cannot find one). Through her death, he is restored to a proper position as the guardian and savior of his daughter's young female sexuality. While this is an accurate interpretation, it is not a complete one. Beth's death is also needed to fulfill the biopolitical desire to achieve equilibrium that protects the security of the population from internal dangers. By disposing of Beth and implying that she was justly punished for her transgression, the pandemic is made to make sense. A seemingly disordered and unregulated world full of rioting, trash, and mass graves still makes sense in its biopolitical decisions of making live and letting die. It is what Fernandes (2004) calls a "double-mirroring," where the modern state labors, like the immune system, to distinguish the self from the non-self. The healthy carrier is thus "a danger to the body politic not because she is a silent carrier of deadly 'germs'; but because she is a 'border figure': Her existence between illness and health, between citizenship and exile defies conventions and authority, disrupting the state's ability to recognize and construct the self" (p. 198). Media narratives serve this very purpose—they make the world make sense.

In an exchange between a Homeland Security official and Dr. Ellis Cheever (Laurence Fishburne) of the CDC, the official tries assess the probability that this virus is a terrorist plot. He asks Cheever, "Is there any way someone could weaponize the bird flu? Is that what we're lookin' at?" Cheever replies, "Someone doesn't have to weaponize the bird flu. The birds are doing that." While amusing, the exchange reminds us that biopolitical governance is first and foremost about accessing and regulating risks. As Elbe (2008) argues, risk is a biopolitical rationality, "for not only does the language of risk accompany various political strategies that seek to manage collective population dynamics, but it is also the language of risk that enables these collective dynamics, including overall levels of disease, to be governed at the level of population" (p. 192). Therefore, in order to further investigate the nature of biopolitical regulation and security in the age of pandemics, I turn my attention to risk society.

Risk Society

In his seminal work *Risk Society*, Ulrich Beck (1992) argues that modernization has brought an emergence of society bounded by risk. He defined risk as "a systematic way of dealing with hazards and insecurities induced and introduced by modernization itself" (p. 21). To Beck, risk was a necessary condition of existence in modernity and the globalized world. It is also a response to a certain future that is to be prevented. In that sense, risk is always already future-oriented, its consciousness lies in the future, not the present. Beck writes, "The actual social impetus of risks lies in the *projected dangers of the future*....In the risk society, the past loses the power to determine the present. Its place is taken by the future" (p. 34). However, as the global world order took over the nation-state as the dominant organizational imperative, the nature of the future has changed as well. No longer contained within the static boundaries of the nation-state, the future has become disassociated from particular attempts to secure or fix its emergence. As Beck and Levy (2013) argue, those new horizons of future expectations are connected to the global diffusion of risk iconographies. In other words, as the future became global, it has become diffused, unpredictable and uncontained within specific sets of topologies, both special and temporal. It has also become resistant to previous guidelines put in place to avoid a particular catastrophe. Beck and Levy (2013) write:

> Modern collectivities are increasingly occupied with debating, preventing and managing risks. Unlike earlier manifestations of risk characterized by daring actions or predictability models, global risks cannot be calculated or predicted anymore. Consequently, more influence accrues to the perception of risk, largely constructed by media representations of disasters, which are mediat(iz)ed through the recasting of these temporal registers. Disasters conventionally signify interruptions. In contrast, in the context of an increasingly interconnected world, they have become limiting cases, challenging the taken-for-granted spatial assumptions of nationhood and its attendant methodological nationalism. Underwriting this proposed reconceptualization of temporalities then is the apprehension of global risks as the anticipation of (localized) risks. (p. 7)

To apprehend global as the anticipation of the local echoes the do-good model of globalization "Think global, act local," but also ensures their mutual emergence (Michael & Rosengarten, 2012). The narratives of pandemic prevention put an emphasis on any local virus, infection, or disease as a potentiality for global ruin. A common headline in local, national, and international news emphasizes the global danger of a local threat, and vice versa. Everything matters. As I illustrate in this chapter, much of the media coverage of SARS or avian flu focuses on how an entity in a local village in the middle of jungle/mountains/forest can potentially bring down the globe. It was a bat and a pig near Hong Kong that almost brought down the world in *Contagion*. Everything and anything can be a potential catastrophe. This is important for two reasons. First, it alters topologies and communities associated with the global and the local, with the Empire and the nation-state. Beck and Levy (2013) argue that there are "risk collectives" that emerge out of the topological diffusement of future and associated risk:

> In the absence of a dominant narrative about the future, global risk frames structure how national experiences are informed by global expectations and how global experiences are shaping national expectations. Perceiving the future through the prism of risk perceptions reveals how representations of catastrophes of various kinds (e.g. ecological, human rights) are challenging the ontological security once provided by the temporal narratives of nation-states. However, the result of these developments is not some pure normative cosmopolitanism of a world without borders. Instead, these risks produce a new 'impure' cosmopolitanization—the global other is in our midst. What emerges is the possibility of 'risk collectivities' which spring up, establish themselves and become aware of their cosmopolitan composition—'imagined cosmopolitan collectivities' which might come into existence in the awareness that dangers or risks can no longer be socially delimited in space or time. (p. 10)

If risks can no longer be fixed in space or time, if the best we can do is conceptualize "risk collectives," then we have to constantly anticipate a catastrophe. Therefore, we are now living in a risk culture (Adam, Beck & Van Loon, 2000). While Beck (1992) argued that a risk society is a catastrophe society, he later corrected that point to emphasize that risks are never done, they are anticipated (Beck, 2006). He writes:

> Risk does not mean catastrophe. Risk means the anticipation of catastrophe. Risks exist in a permanent state of virtuality, and become "topical" only to the extent that they are anticipated. Risks are not "real," they are "becoming real" (Van Loon, 2000). At the moment at which risks become real—for example, in the shape of a terrorist

> attack—they cease to be risks and become catastrophes. Risks have already moved elsewhere: to the anticipation of further attacks, inflation, new markets, wars, or the reduction of civil liberties. Risks are always events that are threatening. Without techniques of visualization, without symbolic forms, *without mass media, etc., risks are nothing at all* [emphasis added]. (Beck, 2006, p. 333)

And in order to anticipate risks, we have to be able to symbolize and imagine them. Therefore, to bring me to the second point, the mechanisms of visualization become important to the risk society.

Van Loon (2000) argues that Beck's theorization of risk society reserves a significant space for the role of media in the contemporary world. Beck (1992) writes, "[A]s the risk society develops, so does the antagonism between those afflicted by risks and those who profit from them. The social and economic importance of knowledge grows similarly, and with it the power over the media to structure knowledge (science and research) and disseminate it (mass media). The risk society in this sense is also the science, media and information society. Thus new antagonisms grow up between those who produce risk definitions and those who consume them" (p. 46). Cottle (1998) explains that Beck's argument clearly privileges the mass media as a site for social construction of risks, therefore connecting the risk society to the study of the social construction and representation of social problems. Moreover, global "mediat(iz)ation" of risks contributes to the future expectations (Beck & Levy, 2013). As argued above, the globalization of potential disasters diffuses representations of risk; therefore, the media becomes important in focusing any perception of risk. As Beck and Levy (2013) argue, "The more obvious it becomes that global risks cannot be calculated or predicted, the more influence accrues to the perception of risk. What is perceived as dangerous is not only a function of cultural and social contexts but also of an issue's career of media representation and social recognition" (p. 18). It is in this aspect that the risk becomes a discursive proposition to be disputed, refuted, and/or accepted. This also helps to distinguish between risk and moral panic. Ungar (2001) argues, "[M]oral panic is constituted by a relatively small pool of mostly familiar threats, or variations on a theme. The risk society is constituted by a vast number of relatively unfamiliar threats, with new threats always lurking in the background. Research on moral panic generally takes a top-down approach to claims-making....Risk society issues do not generally fit a top-down model. In short, moral panic has conventionally focused on social control processes aimed at the moral failing of dispossessed groups.

Risk society issues tend to involve diverse interest groups contending over relatively intractable scientific claims" (pp. 276, 277). Therefore, risk society is more in line with Foucault's argument on biopolitics and biosecurity of the milieu discussed above.

Pandemics are definitely risks. But the nature of pandemics lends itself well to the narratives of the global risk society as well. Beck (2006) outlines three features that shape the perception of global risk:

> The theory of world risk society maintains, however, that modern societies are shaped by new kinds of risks, that their foundations are shaken by the global anticipation of global catastrophes. Such perceptions of global risk are characterized by three features:
>
> 1. De-localization: its causes and consequences are not limited to one geographical location or space, they are in principle omnipresent.
> 2. Incalculableness: its consequences are in principle incalculable; at bottom it is a matter of 'hypothetical' risks, which, not least, are based on science-induced not-knowing and normative dissent.
> 3. Non-compensatibility: the security dream of first modernity was based on the scientific utopia of making the unsafe consequences and dangers of decisions ever more controllable; accidents could occur, as long as and because they were considered compensatible.…Not only is prevention taking precedence over compensation, we are also trying to anticipate and prevent risks whose existence has not been proven. (pp. 334–335)

In the rest of the chapter, I examine how biosecurity of population, biopolitics of milieu, and anticipatory nature of risk play out in media narratives of avian flu and SARS.

Avian Flu

In 1918, the bird flu killed fifty million people because it became transmissible between humans. A 2006 NOVA documentary segment titled *Pandemic Flu* (Fine, 2006) argues that the collective worldwide bird population produces a trillion unknown viruses. Furthermore, it only takes one "mistake" in the structure of any of these viruses to enable human-to-human transmission. But if the scientists do not know where in the viral code the transmission "mistake" is located, they cannot possibly predict the probability of infection or transmission. This still makes human-to-human transmission highly improbable. But this "mistake" did occur in 1918. Therefore, the documentary argues, there is a danger, and we simply do not know if the bird flu will be dangerous to humans tomorrow, or the next year, or decades from now (Fine, 2006). In an article in *The New Yorker* on bird flu in Thailand, Scott Dowell, the director of the Thailand office of the International Emerging Infections Program, which was established by the CDC in 2001, reiterates the same point: "The world just has no idea what it's going to see if this thing comes.... When, really. It's when. I don't think we can afford the luxury of the word 'if' anymore. We are past 'if's.' Whether it's tomorrow or next year or some other time, nobody knows for sure. The clock is ticking. We just don't know what time it is" (Specter, 2005). These examples summarize the mediated discursive construction of avian flu (H5N1) as an always already-future pandemic—a danger that is always coming and always possible, no matter the probability. As such, the mediated construction of the avian flu narrative is based within the discourse of risk society and its dependence on the future as a lived experience of the present. Therefore, I argue that the avian flu is an anticipatory pandemic—it is always in the process of becoming—its danger is always future perfect.

Adams, Murphy, and Clarke (2009) argue that a regime of anticipation is an epistemic and ontological orientation to time, where one is asked to inhabit the future. Since the future is always possible and always uncertain, anticipation "gives speculation the authority to act in the present" (p. 249). The affective elements of future risk become important political tools as "anticipatory modes enable the production of possible futures that are lived and felt as inevitable in the present, rendering hope and fear as important political vectors" (p. 248). Risk then becomes a commodity to invest into as a protection against the future. This, according to Adams, Murphy, and Clarke (2009), produces risk subjects, whose lives are organized through a perpetual state of future emergencies: "Risk subjects are produced as a formation of capital emerging in acts of insurance in a state of perpetual precariousness. Anticipating risk means embodying risk as a sensibility for organizing one's life living at risk" (p. 254). Anticipation is, therefore, a key element in Beck's (1992) incalculableness and noncompensatibility—when risks are incalculable and noncompensable, then, as Beck (2006) argues, the principle of precaution essentially functions through anticipation. Anticipation becomes a tool of prevention—the message is that if we anticipate something, we can prevent it. However, as Adams, Murphy, and Clarke (2009) argue, anticipation is a necessary condition of existence in an economy where "anticipation create[s] spaces for 'ratcheting up' our technologies, economies and politics in response to our urgent need to be prepared, such as injunctions to 'grow' economies by expanding anticipation into new domains and registers" (p. 258). For example, in the report accessing the risks of H5N1 for Spain, Rickard Sandell (2006), senior analyst, demography & population, Elcano Royal Institute, describes the two possible outcomes of avian flu:

> (1) The virus never mutates and, hence, there is no immediate threat of a pandemic; and (2) At some point in the future the virus acquires human-to-human transmission capacity—through either (a) an exchange with a human influenza virus or (b) through gradual adaptation. However, even if H5N1 does not cause a human influenza pandemic, another "new" emerging avian influenza virus could possibly do so in the course of this century.... If the virus were to suffer a transformation, this would almost certainly mark the start of a pandemic, largely because the H5 virus subtype has never circulated among human beings. The vulnerability or susceptibility of the world's population to a mutated H5N1 would therefore be universal. (Sandell, 2006, pg. 3)

The BBC Horizon program titled "Pandemic" (Leonard, 2006), which aired in November 2006, tells a story of what could happen if the avian flu mutates to human-to-human transmission. The program seamlessly transitions from the real footage of avian flu trackers and scientists to a dramatized portrayal of the human avian flu pandemic featuring actor portrayals of patient zeros, grieving relatives, and government officials. It is often hard to tell when the present reality ends and the dramatized future begin. Either way the news is not good. The program portrays the future pandemic as a dystopian land where the young die first, the hospitals must decide who lives and who dies—or in biopolitical terms, make live and let die—the economy grinds to a halt, and there is not enough space to bury the dead. All of this is portrayed as an anticipatory outcome of the human avian flu pandemic.

The program starts with the color red spreading over the map of the United Kingdom. This is interspersed with screams, masks, and images of a virus floating through blood. The narrator asserts, "Something that doesn't yet exist is posing a threat to the entire world. When it arrives, no one will be safe." Dr. Poland—the director of Mayo Vaccine Research Group—extrapolates that "if you were a terrorist wanting to design a biologic weapon, you couldn't do better than designing a virus like this. This is really nature's bioterrorism". Much like *Contagion*, the joke is that nature is already weaponized and ready to terrorize us with its unpredictability. Therefore, it is the purpose of biopolitical governance to assess and regulate risks, rather than foreclose them. The claim to the virus's intent and immorality is confirmed by Dr. Roberts, a principal scientist at the National Institute for Biological Standards and Control (NIBSC): "The human population has never been faced with such a virus before. This is an utterly evil virus." Over images of airport chaos, cancelled flights, and armed military forces, the narrator continues, "The virus will be a mutant, humanized strain of bird flu. When it appears, it could kill millions and devastate the global economy."

The program then shows us an abandoned London and a fabricated newspaper headline "50,000 UK DEAD." The narrator warns us:

> The world's once-busy cities are eerily silent. Only 40 percent of the workforce is actually working. The death toll is rising, hitting the young and fit particularly hard. Public transport has all but disappeared, schools are closed, and public gatherings have been banned. Human bird flu has spread to all parts of the globe. This vision of the future is not science fiction; it is based on the latest scientific research, which informs government policy across the globe. Contingency plans for pandemic flu predict millions of deaths, economic meltdown, and society in chaos. This film is a glimpse of the next pandemic. Using the latest scientific research, we follow the deadly virus and discover how tiny mistakes in its DNA will spell disaster for the human race.

While the program presents that which *could* happen, it implies that which *will* happen. In such terms, it positions anticipation as reality and, to follow Beck's (1992) argument, the future risk becomes a foundation for present behavior. If something that does not yet exist is posing a threat to the entire world and, when it arrives, no one will be safe, then all that is left to do in the present is to anticipate future risks. Therefore, the anticipation becomes a moral economy; a way of life and a way of relating to the world. The program presents the hypothetical as the actual—the lines are blurred and the dramatization is seamlessly integrated with documentary footage. The program shows us what it is like to live in the future so that we can be afraid in the present. The footage of the hypothetical start of this future pandemic begins in Phnom Penh, Cambodia, where, according to the narrator something unwittingly bad is about to take place:

> Twenty-four-year-old laborer Eve Chhun could be any one of millions of migrant workers scattered across the region. He is making the long journey home to visit his family in the north of the country. Although he doesn't know it yet, Eve Chhun is about to become a vital part of H5N1's next step on the road to world domination. It will be the last time that Chhun makes the journey north. What is about to happen over the next few days in a remote part of Southeast Asia will have devastating consequences for every one of us.

Here, the program creates a fictional event in an existing space while tapping into the fears of the global infected Other. We are asked to relate to the possible human avian pandemic as it might occur—the actions of those outside of the Western world become anticipated and unpreventable. As Abeysinghe and White (2011) suggest, "Preparation around the threat of avian influenza reflects perceptions of the globalized nature of infectious disease, the individualised awareness of risk, and conceptions of the boundary of the social body and subsequent blaming of the 'Other'" (p. 313). Here our visualization of the infected Other is based in an anticipatory reality—a space where the Other must be confined—since his/her Otherness would be diminished otherwise. In other words, in order for the Other to maintain his/her Otherness in the present, he or she must remain relegated to the anticipatory, or emergent, space of future threats. Fernandes (2004) argues that the discourse of a global response to an outbreak enacts and unmasks the discourse of the absence of presence, or: "The bio-geographical provenance, the attribution of place to disease enabled by the primitive trope, captures the flows of diseases within a rigid discursive frame that incites a border creating terror. In marking emergent diseases as pre-modern presences, the West exteriorizes the historicopolitical and geographical loci of superbugs....More importantly, by locating the origin of superbugs elsewhere, the West creates the condition of possibility for a global capture that arrests globalization's destabilizing flows" (p. 203).

Another dilemma is to how to maintain the anticipation of a future catastrophe in the face of mitigating present factors. Beck (2006) argues that when risks become real, they cease to be risks. Media portrayals of future catastrophes then become important in keeping risks alive through visualizations of simultaneously occurring and non-occurring events. I argued above that risk must occupy a place between the actual and the virtual in order to remain in the popular imagination. *Pandemic* asserts that while, in the actual, only 151 people have died of H5N1 (out of 256 people infected) and that the virus remains hard to catch, in the virtual, all of that could change in just one or two mutations that would allow for the airborne virus to travel from human to human. While it is not clear from the program how easy it is for a virus to mutate—and a chance that just the right "mistake" will be made—it is clear that the very possibility of an occurrence allows for the documentary to walk a fine line between the virtual and the actual. In the virtual, or the imaginary, Chhun's neighbor is shown handling a slaughtered chicken, and in the next moment, according to the narrator, "The mutation can occur that will equip avian flu for domination of the human world. Deep in the lungs of Chhun's neighbor, the fatal change has occurred. The new virus is now armed. It and its billions of offspring can now attack the ordinary human tissue of the nose and throat." In the actual though, "The reason it hasn't been infecting millions of people is because this H-protein right now cannot attach very easily to human cells and cannot spread from one human to another." Here, the otherness of the mutation also matters. Fernandes (2004) writes, "It is, however, to the inherent mobility of pathogens, to their potential for smoothing spaces and leveling differences that the 'wall of disease' reacts. The quarantining of the cultural and geographic Other within a global epidemiological map negates the possibility of an immunological species-being" (p. 204).

The anticipatory space occupied by risk is also maintained in *Pandemic* through a computer simulation of the entire U.S. population. According to the narrator, "All 281 million U.S. citizens are represented in the computer model. Ages, jobs, family status are all taken into account to predict how likely someone is to catch and spread the disease." Then, "When the scientists set their virtual flu virus free in the world they had created, the results were far-reaching and devastating....In just three months, the entire country was overrun. The sea of red dots leave very little to the imagination. The message was clear: the U.S. is just as susceptible as anywhere else. Once the virus arrives in any country, it's only a matter of weeks before it's everywhere." The simulation is represented as an actual and possible risk. These tentative "could happen" spaces are produced through visualization and narrative and encompass everything from vaccines to hospital equipment. Dr. Wilde speculates:

> In our hospital, we have approximately, at any one time, about 100 ventilators available. In a pandemic, we would still need ventilators for the patients who need them currently. We will, in addition to that, need patients on ventilators who have influenza. Those numbers will quickly overwhelm the 100 ventilators that we've got. There is a very real prospect that we could have somebody who is in need of a ventilator and who will die without it, but we will not have one available and will have to tell the family that we are not able to help their loved one. That will be a very difficult situation for any of us to be in, and I don't relish the thought.

This would mean that the hospitals would have to make decisions of biopolitical governance: make live or let die. The program then introduces an "interview" with a fictional mother of a fictional UK patient zero. She describes panic in the hospital and panic on the streets that follow the introduction of human avian flu to the UK. Dr. Wilde continues:

> I'm not saying that we will have roving bands of bandits attacking our homes—that we will have morgues parked in the streets—that we will have thousands of people dying in the suburbs. It's a possibility, and it's important for us to recognize that that possibility could occur and we need to take prudent steps now to prepare for it.

This is disingenuous—obviously, by saying that something is a possibility one is implying that the event could, in fact, occur. However, should there be roving bands of bandits, morgues parked in the street, and thousands of people dying in the suburbs—which for some reason is more horrifying than people dying the city—what is there to do? How can we prepare for the anticipatory contingency?

The program endorses the approach of a real-life couple from Florida who, should a pandemic erupt, have stockpiled enough supplies for three to four months' self-imposed quarantine. As the narrator states, "Jim and Linda's whole house is a contingency plan all by itself. Everything is in place for the self-imposed quarantine that Jim and Linda are planning for themselves as soon as pandemic flu is confirmed in the United States." Individual preparation and self-imposed quarantine may give a feeling of security and control, except that, as the program portrays in its speculative part of the narrative, it does not work. As a fictional community in the United States is quarantined, it becomes clear that isolation is not in the society's best interests. First of all, the virus spreads anyways, and secondly, if a 40-percent loss to the workforce is already damaging to the national and global economy, a near 100-percent loss would be devastating. The drama *Fatal Contact: Bird Flu in America* (Kerew, Verno & Pearce, 2006)—a TV movie whose narrative is almost identical to the speculative parts of the BBC program—takes place partially in a suburban community in Virginia that becomes infected after a local businessman visits Hong Kong and becomes the index patient. In the film, the governor then quarantines various communities in the state and isolates himself and his family in a bunker under the governor mansion. After the governor's son dies from a diabetes-induced crash, it becomes clear to him that quarantine does not work and, instead, that the focus needs to be on community involvement and volunteer effort. In the film, this response works to lower the rate of death in the state. However, much like "Pandemic", *Bird Flu in America* also states that there is nothing we can do to prevent the pandemic from coming. But these mediated narratives still work hard to create and maintain the anticipatory and affective reality of fear.

One function that these media narratives accomplish is to shift responsibility onto individuals and away from governments and organizations responsible for public health. Abeysinghe and White (2011) argue that in the media coverage of avian flu in Australia, "the concept of individualized responsibility is portrayed through media and government suggestions that individuals and individual businesses are at least partially accountable for their own reaction to the avian influenza threat" (p. 323). The documentary "Pandemic" (Leonard, 2006) also shifts responsibility away from institutions and onto individuals. At the end, the program simply insists that, while we cannot prevent or predict a pandemic, individuals must take responsibility for what is to come:

PROFESSOR DUNNILL: What really concerns me is that, unless there's a good public discussion for this, and some ownership of the problem by everyone, it's going to be much more difficult to preserve cohesion when we get into a pandemic situation. People I talk to simply can't accept that there could be a plague in the twenty-first century.

DR. POLAND: I think until you believe that every tenth person in your community could die next month of a disease they have no control over—until you really believe that, how are you going to prepare for it?

FINAL CONCLUSION: (STAGED VOICE) I encourage you to go back to your counties, your communities. Share the information you have been given today and start the conversations that allow for planning. To start the conversation is really quite simple. You simply need to ask one question: What will we do when? What will we do when 40 percent of our workforce doesn't show up? What will we do when the kids can't go to school but we still have to go to work? What will we do when…? In the answer to that question, you will find your plans.

I argue that these mediated representations of avian flu as a future pandemic risk function to construct risk society as a neoliberal regime where the free market and individuals are responsible for themselves. The most consistent element in these representations of the future pandemic is exactly how alone we will all be when it finally arrives. Perhaps this is the irony of life in a global risk collective. In the next section, I further examine the future and the present of risk in the media representations of SARS.

SARS

The cover story of *Time* magazine for May 5, 2003 was titled "The Truth about SARS" and featured a cover picture of a woman's face covered by a respiratory mask. In fact, images of masks were abundant in Western magazines' SARS stories—in *Time*, *Newsweek*, *The Economist*, and *The New Yorker*, to mention a few. Together they comprised a mediated landscape of representations of Severe Acute Respiratory Syndrome, otherwise known as SARS. They also comprised a representation of global risk acting on a local scale. Beck and Levy (2013 describe this phenomenon as the apprehension of global risks as the anticipation of localized risks. Moreover, the vast presence of masked individuals—on covers of magazines and as documentary and film subjects—emphasized a connection between contagion and proximity, or the danger of life in the biopolitical economy of a risk collective. Here, as Beck and Levy (2013) argue, risks produce an impure cosmopolitanization—the global infected Other in our midst. Lee (2005) argues that the news pictures of mask-wearing people help create the atmosphere of a haunted city. The dangers of city life, emphasized by the SARS narrative, were not simply about an inability to maintain borders in the face of globalization, but rather the ability of a city, as a risk collective, to anticipate dangers or risks, which cannot be delimited in space or time (Beck and Levy, 2013). Representations of SARS within Western media as a scourge of cosmopolitan spaces questioned concepts of "the local" and "the global" as distinct territorial spaces (Schillmeier, 2008). It is SARS' potential as a cosmopolitan phenomenon that imbued it with complexity and social relevance (Schillmeier, 2008). Moreover, Wald (2008) argues that these representations of microbial traffic from primordial rainforest to impoverished cities of the developing world to the cosmopolitan centers serve as a part of the language of disease emergence. Microbes are simultaneously primordial and emergent because "an infection might be endemic to an impoverished area, but it *emerges* when it appears—or threatens to appear—in a metropolitan center of the North" (p. 34).

The media representations of SARS focus on cosmopolitan risk collectives—the pandemic highlights the anticipation of risk as a condition of life itself. *Time*'s story *The Truth about SARS* opens with a warning for the United States:

> So far, the U.S. has been lucky. It has been nearly six months since the SARS outbreak emerged and more than six weeks since the illness spread from its birthplace in southern China to put the world on alert. Yet with more than 4,800 cases in at least 26 countries to date, a disease that has rocked Asian markets, ruined the tourist trade of an entire region, nearly bankrupted airlines and spread panic through some of the world's largest countries has largely passed the U.S. by....But if Americans think that they have dodged the biological bullet, they had better think again....

> Only a few hours drive from Buffalo, NY, or Detroit, just across the Canadian border, a Western city that thought it had done just about everything possible to contain its outbreak keeps losing ground. A few weeks ago, Toronto believed that the epidemic was winding down. Now, with 20 deaths, it's the first place outside Asia to be put on a do-not-visit list issued by the World Health Organization. (Lemonick & Park, 2003)

There are two important tropes highlighted in this narrative. First, SARS has a capacity for total domination, and second, that cities in the United State have to anticipate the same risk as Toronto. In fact, the SARS outbreak in Toronto, while only resulting in about four hundred cases and forty deaths (less than .02% of population were infected), has been a major story throughout SARS media coverage. Of course, as discussed throughout this chapter, this symbolizes a colonial perspective of pandemic media coverage. But it also accentuates the perceived vulnerability of cities as centers of "impure" cosmopolitanization. These themes are picked up and reproduced throughout the media in such programs as made-for-TV movie *Plague City: SARS in Toronto* (Scott, Slan & Wu, 2005). A fictionalized account of actual events prior to and during the outbreak, *Plague City* illustrates "impure cosmopolitanism," or "the importance of global cities not only as central agents in globalizing processes but also as powerful centers of infection that diffuse infectious diseases on a global scale" (Schillmeier, 2008, p. 183). The film starts with an overview of the problem: "On February 23, 2003 a mysterious, deadly virus landed in an unprepared cosmopolitan city, Toronto. This is the story of how close Toronto came to becoming the center of the twenty-first century's first pandemic." It continues to portray how SARS become a pandemic, which highlighted the nature of risk in a cosmopolitan setting. In the film, every new revelation about SARS is accompanied by an ominous view of Toronto's skyline, busy cosmopolitan streets, and other significations of a daily city life. A doctor in charge of SARS research in Toronto equates battling the virus to laying siege to a city. Throughout the film, SARS is discussed as a challenge to biosecurity and the governance of a cosmopolitan population. Closely resembling a scene in *Contagion*, a conversation between Dr. Neville, played by Rick Roberts, and Canada's deputy minister underscores calculation of risk in the system of biopolitical governance:

> DEPUTY MINISTER: There are other factors to be considered here. This city has already lost millions of dollars. We are rolling back taxes on hotels and restaurants, and yet the downtown area still looks like a ghost town. The last thing we need is to get

people panicking again. So before we unleash a witch hunt against the Filipino community, we need to make sure that going public is the best thing for the health of the city.

DR. NEVILLE: NO. We cannot sacrifice lives for economics here! Have you ever seen a person choked to death because their lungs don't work anymore?

DEPUTY MINISTER: Have you ever seen a family on the street because their livelihood is gone?

In fact, the media's framing of dangers that SARS poses to cosmopolitan entities were often done in stark financial terms. The *Time* article summarizes:

> With fewer than 300 known SARS deaths so far, the worldwide toll is tiny...but if SARS continues to spread, its numbers could skyrocket. Its overall death rate of about 6% is far lower than that of AIDS, Ebola, or malaria, but if enough people catch the illness, even a low rate could cause a catastrophe. The financial toll, meanwhile, is already catastrophic....All told, says WHO, the global cost of SARS is approaching $30 billion.

In other words, while SARS' life-threatening impact might be low, the risk lies in cost-potential and contingency of damage to the global economy. It is worth being reminded here that, as Dillon (2008) argues, "[T]he history of the emergence and operationalization of risk has therefore always been situated at the intersection of capital and rule. Rule seeks to secure governability. Capital seeks to profit. Risk combines the two in posing and securing subjects of self-rule not simply in conditions of uncertainty but in terms of measuring their exposure to contingency financially" (p. 320).

Therefore, while, as the article in *The New Yorker* underscores, pandemic diseases are much less economically destructive than endemic diseases (Surowiecki, 2003), the ability of a collective to anticipate and predict risks carries immediate economical and political costs not easily evident in a collective already living with an endemic disease. Wallis and Nerlich (2005) write that the most common metaphor of the UK media's coverage of SARS was, in fact, control. They write that these metaphors "tactically validated a more politically and economically moderate approach. In descriptions of global or local situations, these significantly outweighed uses of the Killer, Natural Disaster, and Bodily Struggle metaphors. Reports of governments' and international organizations' actions thus framed the disease as a problem, crisis or disaster. SARS was successively a 'major problem,' 'spreading out of control,' or already 'out of control'" (p. 2636).

The anticipatory financial ramifications of SARS show the difficulty in planning for the contingency of risks in the age of globalization. While endemic diseases might be more costly overall, they are already anticipated expenses. They are present, not future risks. Their costs are not a test of a collective's ability to manage and secure the future. The unexpected emergent diseases accentuate the noncompensatibility of risks in the global world, whereas the new quality of threats accentuates the principle of prevention over that of compensation. As *Plague City* insists, the constantly changing nature of the global sphere can be mapped onto the changing nature of the disease itself. A change in one leads to an irrevocable change in the other:

DEPUTY MINISTER: What does this mean in terms of controlling it?

DR. NEVILLE: Well, you know why there's no cure to the common cold? The coronavirus loves to mutate. It replicates fast. It picks up pieces of other viruses.

WESTON: With constant change it's almost impossible to control.

DR. NEVILLE: Yeah. I mean, imagine if it merges with something as contagious as smallpox. I mean, you've got the deadliness of SARS with the R-nought of smallpox, you know what you got? Plague City.

The Plague City is perhaps an overreach, but, in its coverage of SARS, the media have definitely found the plague hotel. Much like other media coverage, the BBC documentary *SARS: The True Story* (Higgins & Learoyd, 2003) reports that the spread of the disease was linked to a hotel in Hong Kong, ironically called the Metropole—a cosmopolitan infected space where travelers, who have since gone on to take the disease to their respective destinations, once stayed at the same time on the same floor. The Metropole illustrates, in a moment of precision, the potential dangers of metropolitan environments. *SARS: The True Story* puts it simply: "What made this so disturbing is that Hong Kong is a gateway to the rest of the world." What is dangerous about cosmopolitanism is precisely what can make it appealing—diversity, movement, and global influence. The documentary argues that the World Health Organization's contingency plans could not have prevented the Metropole. The mediated narratives of SARS do not focus on the death toll, which was negligible, but rather on unpredictability of cosmopolitan risk collectives. The discourse around SARS reminded the population that while risk can be anticipated—after all, media narratives always state that it was just a matter of time before a virus like SARS emerged—they are not always manageable or controlled. These discourses illustrate the risk and disavow systems of power as inadequate in the securing and governance of the population. The fragility of biopolitics, as a problem of population, is then brought into focus. Much like in the narratives of avian flu, the media reporting featured the theme of self-reliance, which "stressed that the medical system could not cope with the outbreak well, and that the government was not effective in getting things under control. Therefore, citizens had to protect themselves and the community members had to support each other, particularly hospital and healthcare professionals who were warriors in the frontline" (Lee, 2005, p. 264). As the main nurse character in *Plague City*, Amy, played by Kari Matchett, tells her fellow nurses in this speech:

> We have officially been designated a SARS facility. They're moving all of their ambulatory patients out, leaving us with SARS or suspected SARS patients. As you may know, we're in a volunteer work situation now. The choice to work here is entirely yours. The hospital's doing everything it can to provide us with the most up-to-date protective gear, but even so, there's a risk—a grave risk. But, we're nurses right? A lot of us chose this profession because we wanted the opportunity to help people in times of need. This is one of those times. These people need us.

At the end of her speech, most nurses raise their hands to indicate that they want to take the risk and fulfill their duties. Once again, the response to a global risk lies in the hands of a few Western individuals. It illustrates that risk society works as a functioning component of a neoliberal regime where private communities substitute for public governments and where the public good relies on a few people. In the next chapter, I examine the fictional narratives of zombie outbreaks as illustrations of problems of governance of life itself.

· 5 ·

ZOMBIE PANDEMIC AND GOVERNANCE OF LIFE ITSELF

In May 2011, The Centers for Disease Control posted a preparedness guide to a zombie apocalypse on their blog. The blog post proved to be so popular that, in two days, the website crashed (Marsh & McCune, 2011). The blog post read:

> There are all kinds of emergencies out there that we can prepare for. Take a zombie apocalypse for example. That's right, I said z-o-m-b-i-e a-p-o-c-a-l-y-p-s-e. You may laugh now, but when it happens you'll be happy you read this, and hey, maybe you'll even learn a thing or two about how to prepare for a *real* emergency.
>
> In movies, shows, and literature, zombies are often depicted as being created by an infectious virus, which is passed on via bites and contact with bodily fluids.
>
> The rise of zombies in pop culture has given credence to the idea that a zombie apocalypse could happen. In such a scenario zombies would take over entire countries, roaming city streets eating anything living that got in their way. The proliferation of this idea has led many people to wonder "How do I prepare for a zombie apocalypse?"
>
> Well, we're here to answer that question for you, and hopefully share a few tips about preparing for *real* emergencies too! (Khan, 2011)

The CDC also published a graphic novella illustrating basic principles of emergency preparedness using a zombie apocalypse as a simulation. In the novella, a news channel announces, "Several people have been hospitalized after a strange virus began spread rapidly throughout the southeast. The symptoms include slow movement, slurred speech, and violent tendencies" (U.S. Department of Health and Human Services 2012). The CDC and other government agencies are presented as competent and efficient—the vaccine is developed in a matter of weeks and efficiently distributed to safe centers around the country. However, the vaccine does not stop the breakdown of national defenses. At the end of the novella, zombies have broken through military defenses at the safe center where our heroes, Julie and Todd, are hiding. As a zombie gets ahold of Todd, it is all revealed to be just a dream. While the lesson is supposed to be preparedness, the moral of the story is that no matter what you do, zombies will get you (Campbell, 2012)! In fact, Webb and Byrnand (2008) argue that "zombie-ness" resembles "human-ness" in its ability to invade, infect, and dominate:

> Like humans, zombies aren't social isolates—they seem to prefer to live in groups, within built environments; like us, they actively colonize spaces for themselves; like us—at least in the West—they seek to spread well beyond their local region, and to dominate people and places. Consequently, though we do not know their points of origin, we typically come across them in the most ordinary and safe of environments—as our own home ground. Indeed, there is always something 'nearly me' about the monster. This is evident in how easily we are infected with 'zombie-ness:' a mere bite from one of them, or a drop of their bodily fluid into my eye, and I too am become zombie. The transmission of the 'virus' between us and them indicates our closeness: viruses (mostly) travel between like species, and the job of the average zombie seems to be, (a) eat as many people as possible, and (b) infect as many people as possible. So, the story goes, once they have arrived among us, carrying 'some kind of virus,' they metastasize rapidly, devastating cities, decimating population. (p. 85)

Much like a vampire myth, zombies originate within folklore traditions. The term *zombi* derives from Haitian and West African folklore and refers to individuals whose souls have been appropriated by a special category of priest, or *bokor* (Mantz, 2013). These walking dead are based in *vodoun* religion and Western culture has spent significant resources trying to understand their "exotic" origins. When Wade Davis, a Harvard anthropologist, went to Haiti to look for exotic medicinal treatments, he found that a *zombi* person had an actual role in the practices of *vodoun* religion and was rendered a *zombi* through the careful administration of a closely guarded blend of powerful neurotoxins (Bishop, 2006). Davis goes on to describe his experiences in *The Serpent and the Rainbow* (1985). However, even prior to that, Hollywood films were fascinated with *zombi* and vodoun. Films like *White Zombie* (Halperin & Halperin, 1932) and *I Walked with a Zombie* (Lewton & Tourneur, 1943) show deadly repercussions for white people, and especially white women, who decide to visit Haiti and get a bit too close to the vodoun religion. These narratives were steeped in paranoia towards racial "Others" and mysterious "dark" countries.

In the late 1960s and 1970s George Romero reinvented the zombie film genre and introduced zombies as we know them today. In films *Night of the Living Dead* (Hardman, Russell & Romero, 1968) and *Dawn of the Dead* (Argento, Cuomo & Romero, 1978), Romero established new rules for zombies. They were now autonomous, they partially ate the living, and, after the initial outbreak, they increase their numbers by infecting the living (Paffenroth, 2006). More importantly, the causes of the outbreak have become grounded in current social problems, be it the fear of nuclear war (*Night of the Living Dead*) or bioweapons (*Crazies*, Croft & Romero, 1973). As Drezner (2011) argues, the zombie film genre has moved towards an origin explanation that involves viruses, prions, and toxins.

Scholars have also argued that zombie films represent the fear of conformity (Loudermilk, 2003; Paffenroth, 2006). From communism to capitalism, zombie films have encapsulated fears of individuals becoming a brainwashed mass. *The Invasion of Body Snatchers* (Siegel, 1956) exemplified the fear of communism—alien pods replacing Americans and turning the nation into a conformist nightmare that disposes of individuality. In contrast, *The Dawn of the Dead* (Argento, Cuomo & Romero, 1978) is widely recognized as a critique of consumer society, featuring zombies as drooling consumers trying get into the mall. However, these films also adhere to what Priscilla Wald (2008) calls the "outbreak narrative." She writes that *Body Snatchers*—both the original and the 1978 remake—is "a story about a threat conceived as a public-health concern with medical and/or public health personnel responsible for solving the mystery....Epidemiological horror tells the story of that outbreak as the threat of an ecological 'invasion' that produces dangerous hybrids and generates an apocalyptic battle for the fate of humanity. That framework, and the simultaneous terror and reaffirmation that it generates, herald the conventions of the outbreak narrative" (p. 212). The past decade has also seen an "outbreak" of zombie narratives in film, literature, television, and video games. However, it is in zombie films that the geopolitical implications of biosecurity, globalization, and pandemics—all discussed in the previous chapter—have been treated most thoroughly. In other words, zombie films have become an illustrative example of what happens when disease goes global. It is what Drezner (2011) calls the "globalization of ghouldom."

In the academy, then, zombies have become a tool with which to discuss problems of disease, contagion, and governance in the globalized world. For example, Youde (2012) argues that when an outbreak of infectious disease occurs, the international community faces governing tension between using biosurveillance while still assuring human rights protections. He argues that a zombie outbreak is illustrative of the tentative and tension-filled relationship between biosurveillance and human rights. This is the case because

> most depictions of zombie outbreaks portray an existential threat to the continued existence of society and civilization as we know it...as with the outbreak of any novel pathogen, the origins of zombieism are generally unknown at the epidemic's beginning. The novelty of the disease, along with its mysterious origins, complicates attempts to stop its spread or find a cure. This parallels the SARS epidemic—a disease whose origins remain clouded in mystery today....Three criteria demonstrate why zombieism makes an effective tool for understanding infectious disease outbreaks and pandemic preparations. First, the zombie plague passes person-to-person and via intimate contact. While there may exist animal reservoirs, the zombie virus exhibits sustained transmission among humans. Zombieism is not an airborne pathogen. Rather, it spreads when a zombie bites an uninfected person. Most depictions suggest that the virus is highly (if not inevitably) contagious and that zombies are inherently driven to infect others. (p. 86)

In relationship to governance in times of crisis I want to argue in this chapter that zombies exemplify the problem of governing what Giorgio Agamben (1998) calls "bare life," or "the life of *homo sacer* (sacred man) who *may be killed and yet not sacrificed*" (p. 8). Bare life is produced through the state of exception, in which "at once excluding bare life from and capturing it within the political order, the state of exception actually constituted, in its very separateness, the hidden foundation on which the entire political system rested" (p. 9). However, bare life can only be politically contained in the form of an exception—something that is included through exclusion. Therefore, the sovereign state must govern through the permanent state of exception. Agamben (2005) gives an example of modern totalitarianism "as the establishment, by means of the state of exception, of a legal civil war that allows for the physical elimination not only of political adversaries but of entire categories of citizens who for some reason cannot be integrated into the political system"

(p. 2). However, he argues, these practices have extended to other governing regimes, and "since then, the voluntary creation of a permanent state of emergency (though perhaps not declared in the technical sense) has become one of the essential practices of contemporary states, including so-called democratic ones" (p. 2).

One could easily see how the War on Terror, championed by the United States, constitutes a permanent state of exception through which terrorists—*homo sacer*—are included through exclusion and can be killed, but not sacrificed. I argue that a continuous threat of pandemics in the globalized world constitutes yet another permanent state of exception through which the infected bare life can be included through exclusion. Zombies provide an illustration of this point: as Canavan (2011) argues, "The attractiveness of zombie scenarios and simulation exercises as tools for emergency preparedness planning (including, most recently, at the Center for Disease Control) takes on new relevance; we might indeed recast all security-minded operations of biopower as variations on a single, all-encompassing 'zombie contingency plan' to which we are all ultimately subject" (p. 175). In this context, a decade-long transition in zombie films from the living-dead to what Vint (2013) calls the "infected-living" is important as a signification of the passage of *bios* (political life) into *zoe* (bare life). *28 Days Later* (Macdonald & Boyle, 2002) started this trend, which continued in *28 Weeks Later* (Boyle, Garland & Fresnadillo, 2007), *Quarantine* (Dowdle, 2008), and, most recently, in *World War Z* (Forster, 2013). There have even been comedic variations on the genre that feature sentient zombies, including *American Zombie* (Jung & Lee, 2007) and *Warm Bodies* (Stern, Stern, Webb & Levine, 2013). The lesson of zombie media was that we all could become *homo sacer* through a zombie bite or blood contact, inasmuch as zombies arise not from without, but from within and violence is represented not as casting out, but rather as drawing in (Canavan, 2011). In other words, we are not cast out as humans, but rather drawn in as zombies. Zombies, or the infected-living, are included through exclusion, but, as they draw in, they produce spaces, which then become the permanent states of exception. Sharma (2009) argues that as boundaries—in our case between the living and the infected-living—begin to blur, "Bare life begins to 'run amok' establishing new spatial arrangements where bare life/legally protected bodies and the exception/order are caught in increasing zones of indistinction" (p. 136). While Stratton (2011) argues that zombies are a cautionary tale of what happens to those of us from whom the state withdraws its protection, I argue that the real danger behind zombie pandemics is *zoe* turned *bios*, or that the infected-living way of life becomes our way of life. As Canavan (2011) argues, "It is the zombies, not the heroes, who actually best exemplify the Utopian break, the zombies that create an alternative organizing order for the globe: a zombie nation, territorially overlapping with ours, which has the power to hail us as subjects and which also has power over life and death" (p. 202). In fact, the state of exception ushers in a new state of permanence; hence, the difference between an exception and an emergency becomes important. Emergency implies an eventual return to the norm while exception implies a new norm. Patton (2011) succinctly explains this difference:

> Agamben argues sovereign power is constituted not in creating the rule of law that a police force (including health police) enacts, but rather, in having the power to suspend law, to create a state of exception. Agamben believes that this aspect of sovereignty is now a permanent feature of modernity, visibly—but not only—manifest as the camp, a concept he means us to take fairly literally as the spatialisation of the state of exception for transitory incarceration to be managed by the police as an "emergency." In these spaces, laws cannot be broken because the rule of law has been suspended.…It is important to stress the term "exception" to strip the concept of "emergency" from its imbrications in discourses of natural or divine acts, of events outside social constructions. This move requires us to ask who grants the exception, and how is it that the once-exception becomes the normal state. (p. 104)

In this chapter, I analyze recent zombie films *World War Z* (Forster, 2013), *28 Days Later* (Macdonald & Boyle, 2002), and *28 Weeks Later* (Boyle, Garland & Fresnadillo, 2007) as narratives that illustrate the problem of governance in a global pandemic, or in a permanent state of exception. I argue that these films illustrate the underlying geopolitical anxiety of the global pandemic. It is the fear that a pandemic, if it spreads far enough and fast enough, will alter our way of life as we know it, turning *zoe* into *bios*, ushering in a new permanent state of exception, and forever changing the landscape and governance of the world. In other words, we are afraid that a zombie pandemic will usher in a zombie nation.

World War Z (2013)

World War Z (Forster, 2013), a recent film based on the Max Brooks novel of the same name, illustrates how a zombie pandemic becomes a zombie state. Taking place in an alternate present the film treats zombies not as an isolated threat, but as a worldwide plague, which destroys most of its population and alters the geopolitical landscape and nature of governance. The film's opening sequence demonstrates the world as being still basically the same, but slightly askew. A new day dawns, the waves crash on the beach, birds fly, and the sun rises over an idyllic family neighborhood—the camera work shifts and jars, and yet everything appears to be normal. As a train station fills with people off to their morning commute, the film establishes its global setup: different world communities, ethnicities, and airports all starting their day. We hear bits of television news and talk shows wishing us good morning and predicting the weather. Then we hear a snippet, "A virus changes in a way that allows…" which is then quickly interrupted by a talk show. The camera moves to an eerie shot of a beached dolphin with a commentary: "Yet again today another group of dolphins became stranded." Then a news anchor asks, "Are there any real threats?" and a confident talking head responds, "Not at all." Snippets of news indicate that "the police have seen cases of people acting strangely… The UN Health Organization will not recommend travel restrictions." There are shots of international crowds and a news witness report: "On top of the man, beating him, the man is bleeding." Images accelerate, indicating further breakdown of civilization: fumigated buildings, wolves devouring a deer, rotting animal carcasses, bug swarms, and animal attacks interspersed with images of crowds. This opening establishes a zone of indistinction where the lines between *zoe* and *bios* begin to blur and where the state of exception can begin to be establish. As Agamben (1998) explains, a zone of indistinction is the topology of the state of exception where "[t]he state of exception is thus not so much a spatiotemporal suspension as a complex topological figure in which not only the exception and the rule but also the state of nature and law, outside and inside, pass through one another" (p. 37).

The implicit unease, a zone of indistinction, continues through the beginning of the movie as Gerry (Brad Pitt)—a former UN field agent—is stuck in a traffic jam with his family. Everything seems to be normal, but helicopters are everywhere and the radio reports the outbreak of rabies in twelve countries. The uneasiness builds as a cop motorcycle races by and rips a side mirror off the family car. Gerry goes outside to investigate, and there is suddenly an explosion in the distance. People begin to run. The most immediate thought is that this is a terrorist attack. But this is a zombie film. As a cop tells Gerry to get back in the car, a truck whizzes by and runs the cop over. Now it has become obvious that there is a complete breakdown of law and order. There are masses of people running in all directions. Then we see people jumping on other people and biting them. Here, the infected-living draw us in, infringe on our boundaries, and make us a part of their world order. What we are witnessing is not just a pandemic, but an emergence of a new world order.

As Gerry and his family make their way to an evacuation point, Gerry expounds, "I used to work in dangerous places, and people who moved survived and those who didn't…Movement is life." Zombies, or the infected-living, however, move as well. In fact, in *World War Z*, they move faster and with more determination than the non-infected. If movement is life, then zombies are the most alive of all. The infected are living precisely *because* they are a threat (Thacker, 2011). Agamben (1998) makes an argument that the braindead—or *faux vivant*—enter a zone of indetermination in which "the words 'life' and 'death' ha[ve] lost their meaning, and which, at least in this sense, is not unlike the space of exception inhabited by bare life" (p. 164). Life and death are then political decisions rather than truths grounded in a concrete distinction. They are decisions of governance, not absolute determinations. Therefore, to distinguish between the infected and the non-infected living is the problem for governance of life itself.

According to Thacker (2011), multiplicity plagues the body politic. He writes that the multiplicity is constituted by and exists through "its circulations and flows, by its passing-through, its passing-between, even its passing-beyond—movements that are, at least in cases of pestilence, plague, and epidemic, both the constitution and the dissolution of the body politic. Multiplicity is, in these cases, not simply against the body politic in any sort of libratory sense.…In the 'problem of multiplicities' presented to the body politic concept by plague, pestilence, and epidemic, multiplicity is never separate from but is always inculcated within, the problem of sovereignty. Perhaps we can say that multiplicity is the disease of the body politic, or, alternatively, that *it is multiplicity which plagues the body politic*" (pp. 153–154). Zombies, or the infected-living, are not liberators—but rather the bare life, which spills over from and multiplies within a state of sovereignty, thereby challenging the very ability of a sovereign to govern *polis*, or political life. When Gerry travels to Israel in pursuit of the zombies' origin story, he finds a contained environment—Israel has built a wall to keep the infected out. They are letting in everyone else, because "every human being we save is one less zombie to fight". For a while this is the evidence of successful governance—a fast response by the government leads to the protection of life itself and actually achieves peace in the Middle East. Arabs and Jews celebrate with dance and song by the "salvation gates," and a senior official explains to Gerry, "I don't have answers. All we can do is find a way to hide." But zombies respond to noise. Attracted to the loud sound of peace, hundreds of thousands rush toward the wall, climbing on top of each other—a giant wave crushing against the wall. Eventually the infected-living reach the top of the wall and spill over into the city. Israel's defense fails. First of all, this failure demonstrates the ineffectiveness of walls and borders in the global age of pandemics. But much more interestingly, it demonstrates how multiplicity can aggregate and move, and how ironically it can demonstrate Gerry's principle that movement is life. As Thacker (2011) writes, "Zombies are also massing and aggregate forms. They not only occupy the borderland between the living and the dead, but between the one and the many, the singular and the plural. Their massing and their aggregation is not a matter of number, but also of movement.…The movement of such massing and aggregate forms is that of contagion and circulation, a passing-through, a passing-between, and even, in an eschatological sense, a passing beyond" (p. 157).

How do we govern in a pandemic? According to *World War Z*, we do so by becoming the infected-living ourselves. Based on his observations, Gerry forms a theory that zombies ignore those who are terminally ill—bare life ignoring those who themselves may be killed, but not sacrificed. Terminally ill bodies, after all, are beyond governance. Sacrifice only matters if the body is healthy. To test the theory he injects himself with a deadly, but curable, virus. For a bit, he becomes an infected-living—walking in a "zombie" state, his eyes fixed ahead, through a multiplicity of zombies. His body is antithetical to the *homo sacer*: he is sacrificed, but not killed. It seems that the only way the body politic can survive in the infected-living world order is through a sacrificial body, which is still a part of the political order, or *polis*. However, that body must be sacrificed, even if temporarily, in order to be effective. Much like a virus is not attracted to another virus, so death can only be defeated by death.

Gerry's narration ends the film:

> This isn't the end. Not even close. We've lost entire cities. We still don't know how it started. We bought ourselves sometime. It's giving us a chance. There are those who found a way to push back. If you can fight, fight. Help each other. Be prepared for anything. Our war has just begun.

The perpetual motion stands. The governance of a global pandemic, much like the governance of bare life, is a continuous process of inclusion and exclusion. Agamben (1998) writes, "[W]hen life and politics—originally divided, and linked together by means of the no-man's-land of the state of exception that is inhabited by bare life—begin to become one, all life becomes sacred and all politics becomes the exception" (p. 148). *World War Z*, as a contemplation of biological risks associated with globalization, emphasizes the insight that "zombie wars" can give way to the permanent pandemic, where infection becomes a way of life (Gilman, 2010; Saunders, 2012). In other words, it is not an emergency, but an exception.

28 Days Later (2002) and *28 Weeks Later* (2007)

While *World War Z* begins by establishing a zone of indetermination where a zombie pandemic starts to interrupt the usual processes of biopolitical governance, *28 Days Later* (Macdonald & Boyle, 2002) portrays a world firmly entrenched in a permanent state of exception. The film opens with news footage of riots around the world. These are interspersed with videos of brutal violence, police and civilian shootings, and lynchings. Then the audience sees a chimp, constrained to a table and forced to watch these violent images. At the same time, animal rights activists break into the center, called the Cambridge Primate Research Center, hoping to liberate the chimps held there. A scientist catches them in the act and tries to warn against unforeseen circumstances: "The chimps are highly infected, they are contagious; they've been given an inhibitor. To cure, you must first understand. [They are] infected with rage. The infection is in their blood and their saliva". The activists do not heed his warnings and a chimp bites one of them. Within seconds she gets violently ill, her eyes become red, and she becomes infected with a rage virus. She attacks her fellow activists and the virus spreads throughout Britain.

It is now twenty-eight days later. The audience is introduced to the protagonist, Jim, in his hospital bed. He regains consciousness and wanders out of the room into an abandoned hospital in disarray. Jim walks outside into an empty parking lot and then into an abandoned London. As he walks through various historical sites, periodically yelling "Hello," he finds a newspaper with the headline "Evacuation." Then there is a wall covered with the notes of those looking for their missing loved ones. It is there that he sees a postcard with a line from the Bible: "I will be your grave for you are vile. Nahum 1:14." Jim is disoriented and panicked. After he encounters the infected—as those afflicted with the rage virus are called throughout the movie—in a church, two other survivors, Selena and Mark, save him. Selena explains to Jim what has transpired while he was in a coma:

> It started as rioting. But right from the beginning you knew this was different. Because it was happening in small villages, market towns. And then it wasn't on the TV any more. It was in the street outside. It was coming in through your windows. It was a virus. An infection. You didn't need a doctor to tell you that. It was the blood. It was something in the blood. By the time they tried to evacuate the cities it was already too late. Army blockades were overrun. And that's when the exodus started. Before the TV and radio stopped broadcasting there were reports of infection in Paris and New York. We didn't hear anything more after that.

This description shows how a pandemic can overrun the seemingly permanent order of biopolitical governance. Gilman (2010) writes, "For Giorgio Agamben, sovereignty claims the constitutive right to define, control, and, if need be, destroy its subjects by a process in which prepolitical life is captured by a biopolitical regime. Plague, then and now, has the power to reverse these terms. In a state of pandemic exception from (what we ahistorically assume to be) the 'normal' order of things, nature reclaims its sovereignty over life as death's ultimate arbiter" (p. 35). This means that a pandemic does not just create conditions for the emergence of a permanent state of exception, but displaces the sovereign while creating this new permanence. In other words, pandemics change the way the biological relates to the social and the political (Barney & Scheck, 2010). The new permanence is beyond rational governmentality and beyond the sovereign. In *28 Days Later* Jim is shocked that there is no government, because there is always a government:

> JIM: What about the government? What are they doing?
> SELENA: There is no government.
> JIM: Of course there is government! There is always a government! They are in a bunker or a plane.
> MARK: There is no government. No police. No army. No TV. No radio. No electricity.

Later on, Mark tells a story of how his family went to London's Paddington Station in the hopes of getting out of the city. The story emphasizes the topology of indistinction created by the pandemic:

> I remember my dad had all this cash. Even tho' cash was completely useless.
>
> I remember the ground was soft. I looked down and I was standing on all these people, like a carpet. People who have fallen. Someone in the crowd there were infected

> and it spread fast. No one could run, all you could do was climb...climb over more people...And I climbed. I climbed on top of that kiosk. Looking down you couldn't [tell?] which faces weren't infected and which were. I saw my dad. My dad's face...

The suspension of biopolitical governance ushers in a new, permanent state of exception, which then becomes the new norm. As Patton (2011) argues:

> Just like riot laws and anti-terrorism measures, public health laws inscribe the extraordinary procedures to follow when diseases (or rather, diseased persons) get out of hand. Public-health law might even be worse (or the paradigm for the permanent state of exception) because the implication is that the "population" will desire to be protected against its propensity to infect itself. There is a presumption that persons have already abdicated their sovereignty over their own bodies in the case of epidemic disease; they wish to be protected against the infected, and if infected, wish not to harm others....Scientists use the term epidemic to refer to a hypothetical exception to a hypothesized norm, made real. The exception is hypothetical because the proposed norm might have been incorrect, that is, there may have always been many cases of a disease, but unrecognized. The declaration of an epidemic makes that norm real because until an epidemic is declared over, there can be no reassessment of the actual "normal" presence of disease. Thus, from the moment an epidemic is declared, until it is declared over, the hypothesized norm functions as The Real. (p. 105)

Jim and Selena, and their new travelling companions Frank and Hannah, believe that they can recapture the pre-pandemic governance when they intercept a recording from a military base in Manchester, promising survivors food, security, and an answer to the infection. "OMG! Soldiers!" Selena exclaims happily, hoping to regain security lost since the pandemic. However, when they arrive at Manchester, they find an isolated group of soldiers in an abandoned mansion. For them, the pandemic, like any other crisis, illustrates that we exist in a permanent state of exception, where law and order can be suspended at any time, for any reason. As their leader Major Henry West explains:

> This is what I've seen in the four weeks since infection. People killing people. Which is much what I saw in the four weeks before infection, and the four weeks before that, and before that, and as far back as I care to remember. People killing people. Which to my mind, puts us in a state of normality right now.

The sequel, *28 Weeks Later* (Boyle, Garland & Fresnadillo, 2007), illustrates that simply ushering in a new permanent state of exception is an inadequate response to the new organization of life and death introduced by a pandemic. The sequel takes place twenty-eight weeks after the rage virus destroyed

England mainland. After the infected starve to death and the virus is seemingly contained, the U.S.-led military forces allow refugees to return to London. Forming the "Green Zone," a heavily surveyed and guarded territory inside London proper, the military opens the borders for a limited number of refugees to return to that part of the city. Trimble (2010) writes, "*28 Days Later* and *28 Weeks Later* highlight strategies of biosegregation and quarantine as central to the security state's approach to unruly publics and public spaces" (p. 300). Zones of indistinction formed by bare life are contrasted by the regulated and governed military spaces. As refugees reenter the city they are greeted by a friendly train announcement:

> We are headed for the Green Zone, our area of security and reconstruction, designated as District One. District One is located on the Isle of Dogs. Although the Isle of Dogs is completely safe, the surrounding area of London is not. There are a large number of bodies still left to be cleared from the original outbreak of infection. Rats and wild dogs are prevalent, as is disease. New arrivals are reminded, for their own safety, it is absolutely forbidden to cross the river and leave the security zone. You will be joining fifteen thousand civilians who are already resident in District One. As we approach your new home, you will notice a dramatically increased military presence. The U.S. Army is responsible for your safety. We will do everything we can do to make your repatriation as easy as possible. Inside District One, however, we believe you'll be pleasantly surprised. We have hot and cold running water, twenty-four-hour electricity, a medical center, a supermarket, and even a pub.

The refugees are reintegrated into *polis*; they become a part of a controlled space, a new permanent state of exception, which regulates and manages population. The military is confident in its control over zones of indetermination. When the chief medical officer expresses concerns, they are quickly shut down:

GENERAL STONE:	Major. What are you afraid of?
SCARLET:	What if it comes back?
STONE:	It won't come back.
SCARLET:	What if it does?
STONE:	If it comes back, we kill it. Code Red.

The virus does come back and General Stone issues the command to execute Code Red, which, as Scarlet explains, has three steps: "Step one: kill the infected. Step two: containment. If containment fails, then Step three: extermination." Shortly after, the containment measures fail and the military gives up on selective elimination of the "infected." General Stone issues the command: "Abandon selective targeting. Shoot everything. Targets are now free. We've lost control." Elsewhere, I have argued that the call "We've lost control" represents the anxiety behind containing and controlling threats in the post-9/11 era (Levina & Kien, 2010). However, as I argued above, it also serves as a reminder of the state's inability to destroy bare life. A permanent state of exception needs bare life in order to exist; therefore, it cannot destroy bare life. In fact, at the end of the film, the rage virus has spread to the European continent. Much like in *World War Z*, the walls have failed.

The supposed continuation of the permanent state of exception has a lot to do with the nature of this infection, i.e., rage. *28 Days Later* changed the formula of Romero's films, where zombies staggered slowly toward their victims, and introduced the quick-moving infected, or the infected-living. The infected are not technically dead—they are very much alive, and they can be killed much like regular humans without any specific shots to the head. Eventually they die from starvation—consumed by rage, they do not take care of their basic human needs. They do not eat the non-infected, but tear them to pieces in rage. Trimble (2010) argues that these "neo-zombies" "reconfigure citizens as 'infected' by the anxieties and proliferating instabilities of neoliberalism" (p. 300). She argues that "the rage virus" is a symptom of globalization where "terror, insecurity, and rage can be understood as psychosomatic orientations toward unsettling disjunctions between the local and the global—or between national subjects and transnational corporations, terrorist organizations, and global movements of capital" (p. 300).

While it is useful to examine *28 Days Later* as a cautionary tale of globalization gone wrong, I argue that it is even more useful as a tale of disease governance. The infected in *28 Days Later* are the "already dead," a term coined by Cazdyn (2012) in his book on "the new chronic"—a move in medical sciences to transform the terminal into the chronic and a larger move in the global capitalist system to extend "the present into the future, burying in the process the force of the terminal, making it seem as if the present will never end" (p. 7). The already dead, for Cazdyn, are a way to rethink the relationship between life and death in the new chronic system. The already dead "names that state when one has been killed but has yet to die, or when one has died but has yet to be killed" (p. 165). The already dead hint back at the living; they introduce "another temporal aspect: once we understand that we are dead, we then retroactively realize that we have always already been dead" (p. 165). Cazdyn argues that with the symbolic death, our future begins to change as well.

In fact, when Jim, Selena, and Hannah settle into the soldiers' mansion in *28 Days Later*, they realize that, much like the infected, they are always already dead. The answer to the infection is a reimagining of the future in its most primal patriarchal form:

MAJOR WEST:	I promised them women.
JIM:	*What?*
MAJOR WEST:	Eight days ago, I found Jones with his gun in his mouth. He said he was going to kill himself because there was no future. What could I say to him? We fight off the infected or we wait until they starve to death...and then what? What do nine men do except wait to die themselves? I moved us from the blockade, and I set the radio broadcasting, and I promised them women. Because women mean a future.

As Jim fights Major West and the soldiers, he mirrors the infected—he moves fast, acts crazy, and, in the final fight, kills a solider by puncturing through his eyeballs with his thumbs. At the end of that fight, Selena and Hannah attack Jim, thinking he has become the infected, demonstrating how much his behavior resembles theirs. Webb and Byrnand (2008) write, "Jim avoids the infection, but can't avoid or control his innate, personal rage. The effect in either case is practically identical: for all intents and purposes, in the moments of his rage Jim is zombie" (p. 87).

The "already dead" complicate the line between life and death as separate entities at odds with each other. Instead, the already dead "flashes the radical possibility of usurping dominant discourse of life and death and reigniting revolutionary consciousness" (p. 189). Much as Gerry had to become the infected in order to survive zombies in *World War Z*, Jim had to become the infected in order to survive the military regime in *28 Days Later*. In both cases, the infection served as a liberatory tool, and explored what Agamben (1998) calls "the ontology of potentiality," or the potential of being in the world beyond the dichotomy of life and death. If there is a lesson in these mediated narratives of zombie plagues, it is not just that globalization is dangerous. The lesson is that the true danger of a pandemic is that it forces us to reexamine the states of life and death, that it will lead to a reconciliation of *zoe* and *bios*, and finally, that we will not just become the infected-living, but instead the living infected. In other words, we might just enjoy being zombies.

· 6 ·

PANDEMICS AND DIGITAL MEDIA TECHNOLOGIES

Over the last several years, public health services and Silicon Valley companies seriously considered how digital media, and in particular social media, could be used as a tool to fight the spread of pandemics. Digital media prevention strategies focused on harnessing online social behaviors to track pandemics and to distribute actionable, consumer-based, information. In this chapter, I address how digital media construct pandemics as a global problem that transcends the boundaries of nation-states. I argue that, consequently, these technological developments constitute citizens' health in relationship to their online environments and networks in general. I present a theoretical framework that allows for conceptualization of pandemics in the context of network citizenship, which, as any citizenship, constitutes a particular set of loyalties, moralities, affinities, and addictions. The use of digital and social media to overcome uncertainty and the loss of control in global pandemics serves a counterpoint to the chaos of *28 Days Later*, discussed in the previous chapter. If we account for the infected, or rather have them account for themselves, there is no reason to "shoot everyone." Therefore, network citizenship serves as a contrast to the uncertainty of pandemic control in the global world.

Launched in 2008, Google Flu is the grandfather of pandemic-tracking services (Butler, 2013). It relies on data mining of flu-related search terms and works on an assumption that people are more likely to search for flu information when they themselves are sick (Li & Cardie, 2013). According to various studies, its estimates have matched the CDC's data and delivered results several days faster (Butler, 2013). That is not to say that Google Flu is a substitute for the Centers for Disease Control. Google Flu works with the CDC and relies on its data in its own data mining services. The success of Google Flu has shown promise in the use of digital data to track pandemic spreads and has ushered in what some saw as a radical change in epidemiology—"infodemiology" or "digital epidemiology" (Salathe et al., 2012). The hope behind Google Flu is that this new form of surveillance could take flu epidemiology into the business of prediction, not simply tracking (Dhar, 2013). Therefore, as *The Washington Post* argues, infodemiology "might help forecast and track a flu epidemic the way experts monitor the weather" (Ruane, 2009). Digital epidemiology emphasizes collection of data directly from individuals through various forms of digital communication. Salathe et al. (2012) argue:

> As more individual health behaviors and outcomes are shared online, digital epidemiology offers an increasingly clear picture of the dynamics of these processes. With respect to infectious diseases, newly emerging pathogens can appear unexpectedly, spread very rapidly, and be potentially devastating to millions. A consequence of this change in the epidemiologic landscape is that individual behaviors are now at the center of disease dynamics and control. Individual behaviors will play a key role in social distancing efforts as early responses to newly emerging, rapidly spreading infectious diseases. (p. 2)

The follow-ups to Google Flu rely more explicitly on users for information and reporting. Services such as Sickweather, HealthMap, Outbreaks Near Me, and Flu Near You (both apps offered from HealthMap) involve individuals in reporting on their health for tracking the spread of a disease. Sickweather is the first consumer-oriented product to track disease through social-media chatter by scanning social networks for mentions of twenty-four different symptoms (Kessler, 2012). Their smartphone app uses "geosensing" to notify users when they are near an illness report. The alert appears on the smartphone screen "Attention! You are near a flu report". Users can set up alerts for many common infectious ailments, including respiratory illnesses, allergies, flu, and childhood diseases. Right now, information appears to be sparse and vague; since tracking relies on social media, it privileges more affluent areas where people are more likely to consistently use these online services. However the promise is that "soon, before you enter a Starbucks or sit on a crowded city bus, you will be able to know if some people inside have had a fever in the past 24-hours or a chickenpox-ridden child at home" (Woolf, 2013). HealthMap uses online news aggregators, eyewitness reports, expert-curated discussion, and validated official reports "to achieve a unified and comprehensive view of the current global state of infectious diseases" (About HealthMap, 2006). Their smartphone app, Outbreaks Near Me, works much like Sickweather, but relies on HealthMap data, instead of social media, to show outbreaks of infectious diseases such as H1N1. While Sickweather tracks most common ailments and shows even a single reported case, HealthMap and Outbreaks Near Me relies on more established data patterns to indicate trends of infection. However, all of these services work on an assumption that access to online information and the enabling of user participation will lead to better health for users of these services. Clark Freifeld, a co-founder of HealthMap, wrote that "we aim to empower citizens in the cause of public health, not only by providing ready access to real-time information, but also by encouraging them to contribute their own knowledge, expertise and observations" (qtd. in Goldsmith, 2009). In fact, HealthMap's tagline states, "Increased awareness in your world, means healthier world for all."

These developments locate pandemic tracking within the network society and, with it, a system of power relations necessitated by the rise of globalization and the emergence of information technology (Castells, 2000).

> Network power posits that "coordinating standards are more valuable when greater numbers of people use them, and... that this dynamic... can lead to the progressive elimination of the alternatives over which otherwise free choice can effectively be exercised" (Grewal, 2009, p. 4). The central premise of network power is then that "the benefits that come from using one standard rather than another increase with the number of users, such that dominant standard can edge out rival one" (pg. 26).

As a nonlinear power relation, network power operates through regulations of standards as opposed to the enforcement of a sovereign will. A network becomes stronger not merely because of its size, but as a result of more and more participants embracing particular norms, or standards, of being in the network. This does not mean that network power is democratic—as David Singh Grewal (2008) argues, "[I]n this case, aggregate outcomes emerge not from an act of collective decision-making, but through the accumulation of decentralized, individual decisions that, taken together, nonetheless conduce to a circumstance that affects the entire group" (p. 9)—but rather that it is a diffuse system of control and regulation operating through multitude of nodes. Therefore network power is embedded in what has been called a larger "control society," or exercises of modulations that are always relational, always circumstantial, and always mutable (Deleuze, 1995). Network power is therefore a normative and an expansive affair. It incorporates dividend elements, puts them in relationship to each other, and promotes standards that benefit its growth.

The power of the network is in its continuous and constant growth and openness to divergence and difference (Terranova, 2004). As Michael Hardt and Antonio Negri (2000) argue, "[N]etwork power must be distinguished from other purely expansionist and imperialist forms of expansion. The fundamental difference is that the expansiveness of the immanent concept of sovereignty is inclusive, not exclusive. In other words, when it expands, this new sovereignty does not annex or destroy the other powers it faces but on the contrary opens itself to them, including them in the network" (p. 166). As a result, the network incorporates various bodies and identities while encouraging a set of standards to facilitate a normative positioning of said subjectivities in the network. In other words, we might be encouraged to express our difference in the network, but we are also encouraged to be good "subjects" or "citizens" of that same network, and in order to be good subjects of the network, we must connect our well-being to the network's growth and expansion (Levina, 2009). Therefore, network subjectivity is intimately tied to participation in control society.

Digital pandemic tracking emerges in this context. A child of disease control and social media, pandemic tracking exemplifies and proudly introduces a new model of research that depends on cultivation of the network subjectivities of its participants. Sites such as Sickweather and HealthMap promise, and insist on, a global connectivity, which places one's subjectivity in relationship to others in the network. "As people are equipped with more knowledge and awareness of infectious disease, the hope is that they will become more involved and proactive about public health," argues John Brownstein, a HealthMap and Flu Near You co-founder and assistant professor in the Children's Hospital Informatics Program (CHIP) (Harmon, 2009). Clark Freifeld concurs: "It's about empowering citizens in the cause of public health to both provide them with information and allow them to contribute information to share with others" (Madrigal, 2009).

In his essay *The Postscript on Control Societies*, Gilles Deleuze (1995) writes that control societies can be best understood in terms of networks, where individuals (or "dividuals" as Deleuze calls those living in control societies) are never done, never finished—but are continuously moved from one node to another and, as Deleuze posits, the function of control is to collect, direct, and distribute information. Information gives control its material existence; it's what makes control matter. Alexander Galloway and Eugene Thacker (2007) contend that protocol—a horizontal, distributed control apparatus that guides formations of networks—functions in computer and biological networks when it directs the flow of information. In that sense, "information is the concept that enables a wide range of networks—computational, biological, economic, political—to be networks. Information is a key commodity in the organizational logic of protocological control" (Galloway & Thacker, 2007, p. 57). Generating information gives networks the capacity to grow, to regulate, and to circulate. This is the underlying logic, or protocol, of the network. It is also a basic tenant of network subjectivity.

Information flows in the network are not inconsequential; they alter topologies, relationships, and identities. Tiziana Terranova (2004) adds that "the rise of the concept of information has contributed to the development of new techniques for collecting and storing information that have simultaneously attacked and reinforced the macroscopic moulds of identity" (p. 34). Unlike knowledge, information is always in flux. Knowledge is reified in institutions, while information is continuously changing and continuously in need of control. Without institutions to give it form, information flows through the network—difficult to fix, difficult to manage, difficult to control. Whereas knowledge generates meaning, one could argue that the more information there is, the less meaning there is (Terranova, 2004). Therefore, the constant movement of information in networks encourages volatile spaces, random relationships, and in-flux identities. In the control society, you are your information. Deleuze points out that "the digital language of control is made up codes indicating whether access to some information should be allowed or denied. We are no longer dealing with a duality of mass and individual. Individuals become 'dividuals,' and masses become samples, data, markets, or banks'" (Deleuze, 1995). Identity constituted by information is identity in flux: it can always be changed and altered. More importantly, it can only be understood in the context of other data. Therefore, in the control society, dividuals can understand themselves only in terms of their relationships to others in the network.

Network subjectivity is the imperative of an information-based control society. It grounds dividual identities in the relational aspect of the network where the self is always connected and managed as a part of the network through collecting and sharing information. Dividual identities and bodies function based on the principle of network power: rule through decentralized relations of sociability. As Galloway and Thacker (2007) write:

> Control in the networks operates less through the exception of individuals, groups, or institutions and more through the exceptional quality of networks or of their topologies. What matters, then, is less the character of the individual nodes than the topological space within which and through which they operate as nodes. To be a node is not solely a casual affair; it is not to "do" this or to "do" that. To be a node is to exist inseparably from a set of possibilities and parameters—to function within a topology of control. (p. 40)

Pandemic tracking is a product of control societies and as such it expatiates the functioning of information systems. It is dedicated to the collection, distribution, and circulation of information about life itself; its project is to generate more information. Its product, the always-diseased body, is constructed as the very definition of a dividual. It is a fragmented and fractured entity—a subject for database information searches, an entity to be classified, and categorized. As Terranova (2004) argues, "The cultural politics of information does not address so much the threat of 'disembodiment,' or the disappearance of the body, but its microdissection and modulation, as it is split and decomposed into segments of variable and adjustable sizes (race, gender, sexual preferences; but also income, demographics, cultural preferences and interests)" (p. 34). Much like the case where any virus in the organism can only be understood in the context of its relationship to other viruses, pandemic data can only be understood in the greater context of data. Therefore, pandemic tracking engages in the practice of surveillance, where disease symptoms are monitored and contextualized within the realm of all surveyed data. Surveillance becomes an important function of monitoring data and establishing patterns of information in the network. Pandemic tracking is therefore a function of surveillance medicine, which, according to Armstrong (1995), moves illness from the confines of the body into an "extracorporal" space. Armstrong argues that, in the twentieth century's surveillance medicine, illness, as a referent external to a population, which could then enter and infect the body, was replaced by relative positions of all bodies. Therefore, surveillance medicine "fixed on these gaps between people to establish that everyone was normal yet no-one was truly healthy" (p. 397). The symptom-tracking tools such as Sickweather or HealthMap establish the importance of treating individuals as symptoms-in-waiting—important information that needs to be discovered and logged. "Feeling healthy" is not an option for users tracked by these apps; every sneeze, every cough is a suspect, a possibility, whether deadly or not, for enhancing the power and the reach of the network. It can be argued that pandemic tracking works as a "surveillant assemblage" that operates "by abstracting human bodies from their territorial setting and separating them into a series of discrete flows" (Haggerty & Ericson, 2000, p. 606). Of course, in the case of pandemic tracking devices, the surveillance is participatory. The users are active contributors of information about themselves and others. This is what Mark Andrejevic (2002) calls "lateral surveillance," not top-down monitoring, but rather peer-to-peer surveillance disguised as data sharing and participation in network society.

Pandemic tracking tools emphasize lateral, or participatory, surveillance as a necessary element to collecting and disseminating information in the network. Clark Freifeld calls these tools "grassroots, participatory epidemiology. In enabling participation in surveillance, we also expect to increase global coverage and identify outbreaks earlier" (Harmon, 2009). Flu Near You explicitly calls on participation with its subtitle: "Is it in you?" Through daily email surveys titled "How are you feeling today?" as well as a smartphone app and an online service, Flu Near You collects information from its users in order to track the spread of the pandemic. The goal is to prevent the spread of the flu pandemic, or "to catch the flu before it catches you" (flunearyou.org). While it is unclear how knowing that there are ten cases of flu reported in my neighborhood is supposed to help me avoid the flu, the advertisement for the service is hopeful that someday, as the network grows, the information will become more and more useful for preventing flu and other pandemics. According to the press, this is the first phase of a series of participatory surveillance tools that allow the general public to submit real-time infection epidemiology data (Zoler, 2013). However, discursively these systems do not just operate as tracking services, but rather as tools that enable empowerment through participation in the network. Elsewhere, I argued that in Health 2.0 discourse, empowerment narrative is used to encourage data-sharing in the network (Levina, 2012). In other words, instead of focusing on social and economic inequalities that render certain groups more vulnerable to disease than others, we enact our political participation through data donation in the network. This is obviously problematic for many reasons, but especially in how it constructs and deploys the category of citizenship. I have discussed citizenship and disease in previous chapters, and these pandemic-tracking tools, much like other tools for collecting individuals' medical data, are clearly steeped in the language of citizenship and duty. As John Brownstein claims, "[W]e are putting the public back in public health" (flunearyou.org). Here digital pandemic tracking tools are juxtaposed with public-health government organizations, and participation in these services is seen as democratizing—network power is a liberator from the institutional power of government organizations (Levina & Kien, 2010). This language of empowerment through participatory surveillance grounded in a neoliberal market economy is seen through varieties of celebratory media coverage of pandemic tracking apps and other health information technology. A recent article in *Wired*, titled "Our backwards government can't keep up with the fast and furious germs of the future," advocates for liberation of the free market to develop drugs based on crowdsourcing of health information through online services (Huber, 2013). The author proclaims:

> The sharing of knowledge doesn't centralize power; it disperses it. With this unique form of wealth, the hard part isn't the sharing; it's finding ways to limit the sharing long enough to give markets the incentive to develop the know-how in the first place. With germ-killing know-how, there's the further problem that indiscriminate sharing quickly breeds drug-resistant germs. These problems are solvable, but not by people who reflexively assume that more free sharing sooner is always better.

These statements intuit that sharing is always democratic, that participation is always liberational, and that surveillance is always beneficial. Here the free market economy is steeped in the logic of network society where data sharing and participatory surveillance grow the flows of information, increasing network power and enabling free enterprise. Mark Andrejevic (2002), among others, critiques these utopian visions when he writes that lateral surveillance is

> characterized not just by the carrot of participation, but by the stick of generalized risk: the need to enlist monitoring strategies as a means of taking responsibility for one's own security in networked communication environment in which people are not always what they seem....[This] aligns itself with a series of strategies for offloading duties of monitoring onto the populace—strategies associated with neo-liberal forms of governance, especially as these are mobilized to address a proliferating spectrum of risks in both the public and intimate realms. (p. 82)

Moreover, these discourses construct the idea of a citizen whose "duty" it is to donate and share information in order to increase the power of the network. In the next section I discuss the construction of digital biocitizenship as a part of pandemic tracking.

Biological Citizenship and Disease Tracking

Biological citizenship has been used to describe an effort by active citizens to recuperate power away from medical and scientific institutions through bottom-up activism and a political economy of hope. Nikolas Rose and Carlos Novas (2005) term this "biological citizenship:" "[A]ll those citizenship projects that have linked their conceptions of citizens to beliefs about the biological existence of human beings, as individuals, as families and lineages, as communities, as population and races, and as a species" (p. 440). They argue that biological citizenship operates within the political economy of hope: a social, political, and economic system that advances the view of biology as mutable, changeable, and malleable. Rose and Novas (2005) posit that the political economy of hope requires an active stance towards the future. It serves as tool of active biocitizenship: fighting against injustices and sufferings inflicted by medical, political, and economic establishments and institutions. Elsewhere, Nikolas Rose juxtaposes biocitizenship projects of the state to those of individuals. While the former emphasized population control and public health campaigns, the latter "produced citizens who understood their nationality, allegiances, and distinctions, at least in part, in biological terms.... These biological senses of identification and affiliation made certain kinds of ethical demands possible: demands on oneself; on one's kin, community, society; on those who exercised authority" (Rose, 2006, p. 133). In these analyses, the economy of hope and active biocitizenship are represented as largely incorruptible enterprises that nobly resist institutional impositions of discipline and power. Moreover, while Rose and Novas acknowledge the growth of biocitizenship communities online—Rose refers to them as "digital biocitizenship" (Rose, 2006)—they do not attribute unique characteristics to online communities, but describe communities forming on the Web and outside it as "moral pioneers—we would prefer to say 'ethical pioneers'—of a new kind of active biomedical citizenship. They are pioneering a new informed ethics of the self—a set of techniques for managing everyday life in relation to a condition, and in relation to expert knowledge" (Rose & Novas, 2005, p. 450). I argue, however, that it is important to move a discussion of biological citizenship beyond the dichotomy of power structures and liberation discourses. The sheer volume of economic, political, and social investment into social media and online biocitizenship communities—as represented here by pandemic tracking—makes it necessary to theorize a new type of digital biocitizenship.

This type of digital biocitizenship functions, not through a linear exercise of deterministic power structures, but rather as constitutive of the social processes of network power. Moreover, the act of citizenship is constituted through collection and sharing of information, therefore facilitating network expansion. Through normative relations of sociability, pandemic tracking websites encourage "citizen" participation, precisely because it is good for the network. As Sheth (2009) excitedly argues, "[B]y contributing so much online content, many people have become 'citizens' of an Internet or Web-enabled social community....Thus, the term citizen-sensor network refers to an interconnected network of people who actively observe, report, collect, analyze, and disseminate information via text, audio, or video messages" (p. 80).

In fact, biocitizenship becomes inseparable from network relational dynamics in which subjectivity emerges. Rose (2006) argues that the languages and aspirations of citizenship shape the way in which individuals relate to themselves and others. In other words, aspirations and languages of citizenship produce subjectivities. However, technologies of production shape the nature of citizenship arrangements and its associated subjectivities. Heath, Rapp, and Taussig (2004) write that genetic citizenship transforms the public sphere as a site for emerging "ethics of care"—a site that can only be accessed through the lens of technosocial relations. Biocitizenship, as produced by sites such as HealthMap, Sickweather, and Flu Near You, is shaped directly by "ethics of care," whereas care for one's well-being is exercised through participation in collective efforts to collect and distribute information online. These digital biocitizens are therefore aware of the value of information in control societies; they know that information makes networks function. Whereas biological citizens are reluctant to share their information, digital biocitizens, trained through social-networking technologies and network subjectivity, are eager to do so. Their citizen duty is to increase the capacity of the network.

Moreover, it is worth noting that pandemic tracking efforts represent a for-profit capitalist investment in the collection and distribution of economic data. In fact, most of the online sites that facilitate ground-up disease tracking are, in fact, start-up companies powered by venture capital. Therefore, digital biocitizenship is the product of a unique economic system made possible by the free market economy, which conceives of individuals who are "free" to sell access to their biological information, greater general accessibility to scientific research, and the emergence of technologies that allow for faster, easier, and cheaper access to biosocial communities. Andrejevic (2002) echoes this point when he argues that a neoliberal regime governs with strategies that maximize "free choice" and "personal responsibility." Such strategies then "rely upon the responsibilization of citizen-subjects to take on the challenges of self-management and risk avoidance through forms of monitoring and rationalization associated with capitalist enterprise culture" (p. 7).

Pandemic tracking and network citizenship produces always-at-risk subjectivities where "the future of threat is forever" (Massumi, 2010). As I discussed in a previous chapter, the anticipation regime positions its subjects in a permanent orientation toward the future. Anticipation therefore is an ontological value. It shows us a way of being a citizen of the future. We overcome the fears of pandemics by inhabiting a state of uncertainty and future possibility: we might be at risk "now," but we are working for the most optimal possible future. Tracking pandemics online does nothing for the immediate present, but it exists as a way of managing the future. Of course, the fear of pandemics is, again, nothing new—but the integration of pandemic tracking with digital and social media participation amplifies this and makes tracking of threats a way of life, a necessity of existence in the network. In fact, fear is then "the anticipatory reality in the present of a threatening future. It is the felt reality of the nonexistent, loomingly present as the affective fact of the matter" (Massumi, 2010). In other words, fear and anticipation are the affective mode of governance made possible by a permanent state of exception, as discussed in the previous chapter. Governing by uncertainty means to reconfigure citizen actions away from the political and toward the social, or away from dissent and toward data donation. John Brownstein said of Outbreak Near Me, "[O]ur app is all about giving people real-time alerts. We didn't develop this to increase fear. It's about helping people arm themselves" (Marcus, 2009). However, this misses the point. While it does me no good to know that there are four cases of flu reported in my zip code in the last twenty-four hours, the service makes me *feel* that I am doing something just by logging in time, checking alerts, updating my status, tracking my data, and engaging in practices of lateral surveillance. This is the affective labor of digital biocitizenship in the network, and while we can agree that this information could help us track pandemics, it is unclear exactly how it is supposed to prevent them. In other words, it is fair to ask what this practice of surveillance is meant to accomplish outside of turning citizens into censors, or as Andrejevic (2002) writes, "The level of supervision, information gathering, and assessment associated with increasingly individualized forms of governance through risk, in short, corresponds to the development of strategies for offloading of the duties of monitoring associated with a panoptic regime onto the distributed subjects of the gaze" (p. 7).

The individualization of risk becomes of paramount importance when we talk about public health. As Lupton (2013) argues, the practices and discourses of digital health individualize health risks. These are then seen as manageable and controllable as long as users adopt appropriate technologies for self-monitoring and self-care. Lupton then points out that these approaches to public health "privilege a rational, 'activated' consumer who privileges health over other priorities, who is familiar with and confident about using digital technologies and who is willing to take responsibility for self-care and preventive health efforts" (p. 16). Or, as Rich and Miah (2009) argue, a healthy cyber-citizen is expected to utilize these new technologies to keep her fully informed. Here, once more the health of the individual is equated to that of the network. Moreover, while social epidemiology and population security seek to collectivize individual risk and put in the social, economic, and geopolitical context (Lakoff, 2007; Lupton, 2013), digital tracking technology, as well as numerous other health-related self-monitoring technologies, seek to individualize risk and put responsibility for pandemic management into the hands of individual users. This is what HealthMap founders meant when they articulated the need to put the public back into the public health. Digital pandemic tracking privileges those areas where individuals are already "activated" to be successful censors and reporters. They already must think of themselves as citizens of the network and of a neoliberal economic regime. Overreliance on self-reporting and lateral surveillance could lead to quicker detection of a disease in California, but longer in Alabama; quicker in Europe, longer in Africa. Public health might not be efficient, but it is nevertheless public. Therefore before we fully jump on the bandwagon of efficiency, we must ask what we lose when public health goes online.

Digital media exists, first and foremost, in a global context. And it is a subject to the same hopes and dreams as other mediated communication. Especially in the face of global crises and instability, we look to the media to either save or doom us all. From Twitter revolutions to the use of the media in pandemic education and prevention efforts, it is assumed that media serves an important part in how we manage and solve global instability. In this book, I aimed to provide a foundation to cultural debates and struggles over the role of the media in the global environment. I argued that from fictional narratives of vampires and zombie pandemics to earnest documentaries and mediated public health campaigns, the media imagines disease and difference as a problem of global flows of information, commerce, and scientific exploration, to name a few. As such, representations of pandemics in the media constitute subjects to the biopolitical regime of governance. We are always already globally diseased bodies. We might just not know it yet.

REFERENCES

Abeysinghe, Sudeepa, & White, Kevin. (2011). The avian influenza pandemic: Discourses of risk, contagion and preparation in Australia. *Health, Risk & Society, 13*(4), 311–326.

About Health Map. (2006). Retrieved from http://healthmap.org/site/about

Adam, Barbara, Beck, Ulrich, & Van Loon, Joost. (2000). *The risk society and beyond: Critical issues for social theory*. London: Sage.

Adams, Vincanne, Murphy, Michelle, & Clarke, Adele E. (2009). Anticipation: Technoscience, life, affect, temporality. *Subjectivity, 28*(1), 246–265.

Agamben, Giorgio. (1998). *Homo sacer: Sovereign power and bare life*. (Daniel Heller-Roazen, Trans.). Stanford, CA: Stanford University Press. (Original work published 1995)

Agamben, Giorgio. (2005). *State of exception*. (Kevin Attell, Trans.). Chicago, IL: University of Chicago Press. (Original work published 2003)

AIDS in Thailand in *Rx for survival. A global health challenge*. (2005). Paula S. Apsell and Larry Klein (Producers). United States: WGBH/NOVA Science Unit and Vulcan Productions

Anderson, Benedict. (2006). *Imagined communities: Reflections on the origin and spread of nationalism*. (Revised ed.). New York, NY: Verso.

Andrejevic, Mark. (2002). The work of watching one another: Lateral surveillance, risk, and governance. *Surveillance & Society, 2*(4), 479–497.

Apted, Michael, O'Conner, Robert (Producers), & Coppola, Francis Ford (Director). (1992). *Bram Stoker's Dracula* [Motion Picture]. United States: Columbia Pictures.

Arad, Avi, Calamari, Joseph, Harris, Lynn, Lee, Stan (Producers), & Norrington, Stephen (Director). (1998). *Blade* [Motion picture]. United States: New Line Cinema.

Arata, Stephen D. (1990). The Occidental Tourist: Dracula and the Anxiety of Reverse Colonization. *Victorian Studies*, 621–645.

Argento, Claudio, Cuomo, Alfredo (Producers), & Romero, George (Director). (1978). *Dawn of the dead* [Motion picture]. United States: United Film Distribution Company.

Armstrong, David. (1995). The rise of surveillance medicine. *Sociology of Health & Illness, 17*(3), 393–404.

Asma, Stephen. (2009). *On monsters: An unnatural history of our worst fears*. New York: Oxford University Press.

Associated Press. (2009, April 27). Israel must call new disease Mexican flu, as swine unkosher. *Haaretz*.Retrievedfromhttp://www.haaretz.com/news/israel-must-call-new-disease-mexico-flu-as-swine-unkosher-1.274932

Auerbach, Nina. (1997). *Our vampires, ourselves*. Chicago, IL: University of Chicago Press.

Austin, Sydney B. (1989). AIDS and Africa: United States media and racist fantasy. *Cultural Critique, 14*, 129–52.

Barker, Greg, Cran, William, Simone, Renata (Writers), Barker, Greg, & Cran, William (Directors). (2006, May 30). *The age of AIDS* [Television series episode]. In David Fanning, Mark Reynolds, & Michael Sullivan (Producers), *Frontline*. United States: PBS.

Barney, Richard A, & Scheck, Helene. (2010). Introduction: Early and modern biospheres, politics, and the rhetorics of plague. *Journal for Early Modern Cultural Studies, 10*(2), 1–22.

Barthes, Roland. (1972). *Mythologies*. New York, NY: Farrar, Straus and Giroux. (Original work published 1957)

Bartholet, Jeffrey. (1996, February 12). A new kind of blood libel. *Newsweek*, 40–41.

Bayer, Ronald. (1999). Blood and AIDS in America: Science, politics, and the making of an iatrogenic catastrophe. In Eric A. Feldman & Ronald Bayer (Eds.), *Blood feuds: AIDS, blood, and the politics of medical disaster* (pp. 19–58). New York, NY: Oxford University Press.

BBC News (2004, December 1st). Brazil to break AIDS drug patents. Retrieved from http://news.bbc.co.uk/2/hi/health/4059147.stm

Beck, Ulrich. (1992). *Risk society: Towards a new modernity*. London: Sage.

Beck, Ulrich. (2006). Living in the world risk society. *Economy and Society*, 35(3), 329–345.

Beck, Ulrich, & Levy, Daniel. (2013). Cosmopolitanized nations: Re-imagining collectivity in world risk society. *Theory, Culture & Society*, 30(3), 3–31.

Bennett, Jeffrey. (2008). Passing, protesting, and the arts of resistance: Infiltrating the ritual space of blood donation. *Quarterly Journal of Speech*, 94(1), 23–43.

Berkman, Alan, Garcia, Jonathan, Muñoz-Laboy, Miguel, Paiva, Vera, & Parker, Richard (2005). A critical analysis of the Brazilian response to HIV/AIDS: Lessons learned for controlling and mitigating the epidemic in developing countries. *American Journal of Public Health*, 95(7), 1162–1172.

Berlant, Lauren G. (1997). *The queen of America goes to Washington city: Essays on sex and citizenship*. Durham, NC: Duke University Press.

Biehl, J. (2004). The activist state: Global pharmaceuticals, aids, and citizenship in Brazil. *Social Text*, 22(3), 105–132.

Bishop, Kyle. (2006). Raising the dead: Unearthing the nonliterary origins of zombie cinema. *Journal of Popular Film and Television*, *33*(4), 196–205.

Blood Type. (n.d.). *Blood Type*. Retrieved from http://www.nrao.edu/~jogle/blood.htm.

Boyle, Danny, Garland, Alex (Producers), & Fresnadillo, Juan C. (Director). (2007). *28 weeks later* [Motion picture]. United Kingdom: 20th Century Fox.

Bradsher, Keith. (2009, April 28). The naming of swine flu, a curious matter. *The New York Times*. Retrieved from http://www.nytimes.com/2009/04/29/world/asia/29swine.html?ref=health

Bright, William (Ed.). (1992). *International encyclopedia of linguistics* (Vol. 2). New York, NY: Oxford University Press.

Butler, Declan. (2013, February 13). When Google got flu wrong. *Nature*. Retrieved from http://www.nature.com/news/when-google-got-flu-wrong-1.12413

Campbell, Andy. (2012, June 1). Zombie apocalypse: CDC denies existence of zombies Despite cannibal incidents. *The Huffington Post*. Retrieved from http://www.huffingtonpost.com/2012/06/01/cdc-denies-zombies-existence_n_1562141.html

Campbell, Peter. (2013). Intersectionality bites: Metaphors of race and sexuality in HBO's *True blood*. In Marina Levina & Diem-My Bui (Eds.), *Monster culture in the 21st century: A reader*. New York, NY: Bloomsbury.

Camporesi, Piero. (1995). *Juice of life: The symbolic and magic significance of blood.* (Robert Barr, Trans.). New York, NY: Continuum.

Canavan, Gerry. (2011). Fighting a war you've already lost: Zombies and zombies in *Firefly/Serenity* and *Dollhouse*. *Science Fiction Film and Television*, 4(2), 173–203.

Case, Sue-Ellen. (2000). Tracking the vampire (extract). In Ken Gelder (Ed.), *The horror reader* (pp. 198–209). New York, NY: Routledge.

Castells, Manuel. (2000). *The rise of the network society* (2nd ed.). Oxford: Blackwell.

Cazdyn, Eric. (2012). *The already dead: The new time of politics, culture, and illness*. Durham, NC: Duke University Press.

Chaudhuri, Shohini. (1997). Visit of the body snatchers: Alien invasion themes in vampire narratives. *Camera Obscura*, 14(1–2 40–41), 180–198.

Chinn, Sara E. (2000). *Technology and the logic of American racism: A cultural history of the body as evidence*. New York, NY: Continuum.

Cohen, Stanley (2002). *Folk devils and moral panics: The creation of the Mods and Rockers*(3rd ed.). Abingdon, Oxon: Routledge.

Community Blood Bank of the Kansas City Area, Inc. v. Fed. Trade Commission, 405 F. 2d 1011, 1022 (8th Cir. 1969).

Corbin, Carol, & Campbell, Robert. (1999). Postmodern iconography and perspective in Coppola's *Bram Stoker's Dracula*. *Journal of Popular Film and Television*, *27*(2), 40–48.

Cottle, Simon. (1998). Ulrich Beck, 'Risk Society' and the media: A catastrophic view? *European Journal of Communication*, *13*(1), 5–32.

Critcher, Chas. (2008). Moral panic analysis: Past, present and future. *Sociology Compass*, *2*(4), 1127–1144.

Croft, A. C. (Producer), & Romero, George (Director). (1973). *The crazies* [Motion Picture]. United States: Cambist Films.

Davidson, Arnold. (1991). The horror of monsters. In James Sheehan & Morton Sosna (Eds.), *The boundaries of humanity: Humans, animals, machines* (pp. 36–68). Oakland, CA: University of California Press.

Davis, Wade. (1985). *The serpent and the rainbow*. New York, NY: Simon & Schuster.

Deleuze, Gilles. (1995). *Negotiations*. New York, NY: Columbia University Press.

Dentzer, Susan. Brazil's survival plan for HIV. *PBS Newshour*. Retrieved from http://www.pbs.org/newshour/bb/health-july-dec03-brazil_7-15/

Derrida, Jacques. (1978). *Writing and difference*. (Alan Bass, Trans.). Chicago, IL: The University of Chicago Press.

Derrida, Jacques. (1997). *Of grammatology* (Corrected ed.). (Gayatri Chakravorty Spivak, Trans.). Baltimore, MD: The Johns Hopkins University Press.

DeYoung, Mary. (1998). Another look at moral panics: The case of satanic day care centers. *Deviant Behavior, 19*(3), 257-278.

Dhar, Michael. (2013, September 19). Flu watchers: How influenza trackers keep you healthy. *Live Science*. Retrieved from http://www.livescience.com/39788-flu-watchers-influenzavirus-trackers.html

Dika, Vera. (1996). From Dracula—with love. In Barry Keith Grant (Ed.), *The dread of difference*. Austin, TX: University of Texas Press.

Dillon, Michael. (2008). Underwriting security. *Security Dialogue* 39(2–3), 309–332.

Douglas, Mary. (1966). *Purity and Danger*. London: Routledge and Kegan Paul.

Dowdle, John (Director). (2008). *Quarantine* [Motion Picture], United States: Andale Pictures.

Dresser, Norine. (1989). *American vampires: Fans, victims, practitioners*. New York, NY: Norton.

Drezner, Daniel W. (2011). *Theories of international politics and zombies*. Princeton, NJ: Princeton University Press.

Duffield, Mark, & Waddell, Nicholas. (2006). Securing humans in a dangerous world. *International Politics*, 43(1), 1–23.

Dulles, Foster R. (1950). *The American Red Cross: A history*. New York, NY: Harper & Brothers.

Elbe, Stefan. (2008). Risking lives: AIDS, security and three concepts of risk. *Security Dialogue*, 39(2–3), 177–198.

Enserink, Martin. (2009, July 7). International agencies try to end flu naming wars. *Science*. Retrieved from http://news.sciencemag.org/2009/07/international-agencies-try-end-flu-naming-wars.

Epstein, Steven. (1996). *Impure science: AIDS, activism, and the politics of knowledge*. Berkeley, CA: University of California Press.

Erni, John N. (2006). Epidemic imaginary: Performing global figurations of "Third World AIDS." *Space and Culture*, 9(4), 429–452.

Fairchild, Amy L. (2003). *Science at the borders: Immigrant medical inspection and the shaping of the modern industrial labor force*. Baltimore, MD: The Johns Hopkins University Press.

Falco, Miriam. (2009, September 11). Stop calling it swine flu! *CNN*. Retrieved from http://thechart.blogs.cnn.com/2009/09/11/stop-calling-it-swine-flu/

Fee, Elizabeth, & Fox, Daniel M. (Eds.). (1988). *AIDS: The burdens of history*. Berkeley, CA: University of California Press.

Feldman, Eric A. (1999). HIV and blood in Japan: Transforming private conflict into public scandal. In Eric A. Feldman & Robert Bayer (Eds.), *Blood feuds: AIDS, blood, and the politics of medical disaster* (pp. 59–94). New York, NY: Oxford University Press.

Feldman, Eric S., Nabatoff, Diane (Producers), & Bigelow, Kathryn (Director). (1987). *Near dark* [Motion Picture]. United States: De Laurentis Entertainment Group.

Fernandes, Jorge. (2004). Ebola takes to the road: Viruses in defense of the nation-state. In Jenny Edkins, Véronique Pin-Fat & Michael J. Shapiro (Eds.), *Sovereign lives: Power in global politics* (pp. 189–210). New York, NY: Routledge.

Fine, Samuel (Director). (2006). *Pandemic flu* [Television series episode]. In Samuel Fine (Producer), *NOVA*. United States: WGBH Educational Foundation.

FluNearYou: https://flunearyou.org/

Fontaine, Philippe. (2002). Blood, politics, and science: Richard Titmuss and the Institute of Economic Affairs, 1957–1973. *Isis*, *93*(3), 401–434.

Fordham, Graham. (2001). Moral panic and the construction of national order: HIV/AIDS risk groups and moral boundaries in the creation of modern Thailand. *Critique of Anthropology*, *21*(3), 259–316.

Forster, Marc (Producer, Director). (2013). *World war Z* [Motion picture]. United States: Paramount Pictures.

Foucault, Michel. (1972). *The Archaeology of Knowledge*. New York, NY: Pantheon Books.

Foucault, Michel. (1978). *The history of sexuality* (Vol. 1). New York, NY: Pantheon.

Foucault, Michel. (1980). Two lectures. In *Power/knowledge* (pp. 78–108). (Kate Soper, Trans.). New York, NY: Pantheon.

Foucault, Michel. (1988). *Madness and civilization: A history of insanity in the age of reason*. New York, NY: Vintage. (Original work published 1961)

Foucault, Michel. (1994). *The birth of the clinic: An archaeology of medical perception*. New York, NY: Vintage. (Original work published 1963)

Foucault, Michel. (2003). *Society must be defended*. (David Macey, Trans.). New York, NY: Picador. (Original work published 1997)

Foucault, Michel. (2007). *Security, territory, population*. (Graham Bruchell, Trans.). New York, NY: Palgrave. (Original work published 2004)

Franklin, Sarah, & McKinnon, Susan (Eds.). (2001). *Relative values: Reconfiguring kinship studies*. Durham, NC: Duke University Press.

Freeland, Cynthia A. (2000). *The Naked and the Undead*. Boulder, CO: Westview Press.

Galloway, Alexander, & Thacker, Eugene. (2007). *The exploit: A theory of networks*. Minneapolis, MN: University of Minnesota Press.

Geffen, David (Producer), & Jordan, Niel (Director). (1994). *Interview with the vampire* [Motion picture]. United States: Warner Bros.

Gilman, Ernest. (2010). The subject of the plague. *Journal for Early Modern Cultural Studies*, *10*(2), 23–34.

Gilman, Sander. (1988). *Disease and representation: Images of illness from madness to AIDS*. Ithaca, NY: Cornell University Press.

Gilman, Sander. (2010). Moral panic and pandemics. *The Lancet*, *375*(9729), 1866–1867.

Girard, Rene. (1979). *Violence and the sacred.* Baltimore, MD: The John Hopkins University Press.

Glied, Sherry. (1999). The circulation of blood: AIDS, blood, and the economics of information. In Eric A. Feldman & Robert Bayer (Eds.), *Blood feuds: AIDS, blood, and the politics of medical disaster* (pp. 323–348). New York, NY: Oxford University Press.

Goldsmith, Samuel. (2009, September 2). Free iphone app, 'Outbreaks Near Me,' helps users Track swine flu. *New York Daily News.* Retrieved from http://www.nydailynews.com/money/free-iphone-app-outbreaks-helps-users-track-swine-flu-article-1.401815

Goode, Erich, & Ben-Yehuda, Nachman. (1994). Moral panics: Culture, politics, and social construction. *Annual Review of Sociology, 20*(1), 149–171.

Gordon, Joan, Hollinger, Veronica, & Aldiss, Brian. (Eds.). (1997). *Blood read: The vampire as metaphor in contemporary culture.* Philadelphia, PA: University of Pennsylvania Press.

Grady, Denise. (2009, April 30). W.H.O. gives virus a name that's more scientific and less loaded. *The New York Times.* Retrieved from http://www.nytimes.com/2009/05/01/health/01name.html?ref=worldhealthorganization

Gramsci, Antonio. (2000). *The Antonio Gramsci reader: Selected writings 1916–1935.* David Forgacs (Ed.). New York, NY: NYU Press.

Grewal, David Singh. (2008). *Network power: The social dynamics of globalization.* New Haven, CT: Yale University Press.

Hagen, Piet. J. (1982). *Blood: Gift or merchandise.* New York, NY: Alan R. Liss.

Haggerty, Kevin, & Ericson, Richard. (2000). The surveillant assemblage. *The British Journal of Sociology, 51*(4), 605–622.

Halberstam, Judith. (1995). *Skin shows: Gothic horror and the technology of monsters.* Durham, NC: Duke University Press.

Hall, Stuart, Chas, Critcher, Charles, Jefferson, Tony, Clarke, John, & Roberts, Brian. (1978). *Policing the crisis: Mugging, the state and law and order.* London: Macmillan.

Hall, Stuart, Evans, Jessica & Nixon, Sean (Eds.). (1997). *Representation: Cultural representations and signifying practices.* London: Sage.

Hall, Stuart, Critcher, Chas, Jefferson, Tony, Clarke, John, & Roberts, Bryan (2006). The changing shape of 'panics.' In Chas Critcher (Ed.), *Critical readings: Moral panics and the media* (pp. 41–49). Maidenhead, England: Open University Press.

Halperin, Edward (Producer), & Halperin, Victor (Director). (1932). *White zombie* [Motion picture]. United States: United Artists.

Hardman, Karl, Streiner, Russell (Producers), & Romero, George (Director). (1968). *Night of the living dead* [Motion picture]. United States: The Walter Reade Organization.

Hardt, Michael, & Negri, Antonio. (2000). *Empire.* Cambridge, MA: Harvard University Press.

Harmon, Katherine. (2009, September 1). Sick app tracks H1N1, other outbreaks near you. *Scientific American.* Retrieved from http://www.scientificamerican.com/blog/post.cfm?id=sick-mobile-app-tracks-h1n1-other-o-2009-09-01

Heath, Deborah, Rapp, Rayna, & Taussig, Karen-Sue. (2004). Genetic citizenship. In David Nugent & Joan Vincent (Eds.), *A companion to the anthropology of politics* (pp. 152–167). Oxford: Blackwell.

Heaton, L. D. (1964). *Blood program in World War II*. Washington, DC: Office of the Surgeon General, Medical Department, United States Army.

Hebdige, Dick. (1993). From culture to hegemony. In Simon During (Ed.), *The cultural studies reader* (357–367). New York, NY: Routledge.

Hier, Sean P. (2008). Thinking beyond moral panic: Risk, responsibility, and the politics of moralization. *Theoretical Criminology, 12*(2), 173–190.

Higgins, Jackie, & Learoyd, Sue (Writers). (2003, May 29). SARS: The true story [Television series episode]. In Jackie Higgins & Sue Learoyd (Producers), *Horizon*. London: BBC.

Hough, Douglas. E. (1978). *The market for human blood*. Lanham, MD: Lexington.

How Cuba Deals with AIDS. (2013). *CBS News*. Retrieved from http://www.cbsnews.com/video/watch/?id=2931465n

Huber, Peter. (2013, November 9). Backwards regulations can't keep up with the fast and furious germs of the future. *Wired*. Retrieved from http://www.wired.com/opinion/2013/11/how-20th-century-law-code-messes-with-21st-century-bio-code/

Huet, Marie-Hélène. (1993). *Monstrous imagination*. Cambridge, MA: Harvard University Press.

Hurd, Charles. (1959). *The compact history of the American Red Cross*. New York, NY: Hawthorn.

Inspections, compliance, enforcement, and criminal investigations (2011). *CPG 230.120-Human blood and blood products as drugs*. Retrieved fromhttp://www.fda.gov/ICECI/ComplianceManuals/CompliancePolicyGuidanceManual/ucm073863.htm

Inspections, compliance, enforcement, and criminal investigations. (2011). *Manual of compliance policy guides*. Retrieved from http://www.fda.gov/ora/compliance_ref/cpg/cpgbio/cpg230-120.htm

Johnson, David B (Ed.). (1977). *Blood policy: Issues and alternatives*. Washington, DC: American Enterprise Institute for Public Policy Research.

Jordan, John W. (1999). Vampire cyborgs and scientific imperialism: A reading of the science-mysticism polemic in *Blade*. *Journal of Popular Film & Television, 27*(2), 4–15.

Jung, Teddy Hoon-Tack (Producer), & Lee, Grace (Director). (2007). *American zombie* [Motion Picture). United States: iHQ.

Kaarsholm, Preben. (2005). Moral panic and cultural mobilization: Responses to transition, crime and HIV/AIDS in KwaZulu-Natal. *Development and Change*, 36(1), 133–156.

Kaplan, Edward. H. (1998, July 1). Was Israel's Ethiopian blood band justified? *CIRA Policy Update*, 1.

Kendrick, Douglas Blair. (1989). *Blood program in World War 2 (Supplemented with Experiences in the Korean War)*. Provided by the Office of Medical History, Office of the Surgeon General/U.S. Army Medical Command. *PBS*. Retrieved from http://www.pbs.org/wnet/redgold/basics/bloodprograms3.html

Kerew, Diana, Verno, Judith (Producers), & Pearce, Richard (Director). (2006). *Fatal contact* [Motion picture]. United States: Sony Pictures Home Entertainment.

Kessler, Sarah. (2012, June 8). Twitter can track disease—can it prevent outbreaks? *Mashable*. Retrieved from http://mashable.com/2012/06/08/social-media-disease-tracking/

Kevles, Daniel J. (2001). *In the name of eugenics: Genetics and the uses of human heredity* (4th printing ed.). Cambridge, MA: Harvard University Press.

Khan, Ali S. (2011, May 16). Preparedness 101: Zombie apocalypse. *Public Health Matters Blog*. Retrieved from http://blogs.cdc.gov/publichealthmatters/2011/05/preparedness-101-zombie-apocalypse/

Kimbrell, Andrew. (1993). *The human body shop*. San Francisco, CA: Harper San Francisco.

King, Jonathan, Polaire, Michael, Skoll, Jeff (Producers), & Soderbergh, Steven (Director). (2011). *Contagion*. [Motion Picture]. United States: Warner Brothers Pictures.

Kinsella, James. (1989). *Covering the plague: AIDS and the American media*. New Brunswick, NJ: Rutgers University Press.

Krisberg, Kim. (2011). New movie puts public health, infectious disease in spotlight: Behind the scenes of 'Contagion.' *The Nation's Health*. Retrieved from http://thenationshealth.aphapublications.org/content/41/7/1.4.full

Lakoff, Andrew, & Collier, Stephen. (2008). *Biosecurity intervention: Global health and security in question*. New York, NY: Columbia University Press.

Lakoff, Andrew. (2007). Preparing for the next emergency. *Public Culture*, *19*(2), 247–271.

Lakoff, George, & Johnson, Mark. (2003). *Metaphors we live by*. Chicago, IL: The University of Chicago Press.

Langer, Carole (Writer). (1993, November 30). AIDS, blood and politics [Television series episode]. In Carole Langer (Producer), *Frontline*. United States: PBS.

Latour, Bruno. (2004). *Politiques de la nature*. Paris: Éditions La Decouverte & Syros.

Latour, Bruno. (2004a). Whose cosmos, which cosmopolitics? Comments on the peace terms of Ulrich Beck. *Common Knowledge*, *10*(3), 450–462.

Lee, Alice Y. L. (2005). Between global and local: The glocalization of online news coverage on the trans-regional crisis of SARS. *Asian Journal of Communication*, *15*(3), 255–273.

Lemonick, Michael, & Park, Alice. (2003, May 5). The truth about SARS. *Time*. Retrieved from http://content.time.com/time/magazine/article/0,9171,1004763,00.html

Leonard, Peter (Writer, Director). (2006). Pandemic [Television series episode]. In *Horizon*. London: BBC.

Leroi, Armand. (2003). *Mutants: On genetic variety and the human body*. New York, NY: Viking.

Levina, Marina. (2007). Cracking the code: Genomics in documented fantasies and fantastic documentaries. In Margret Grebowicz (Ed.), *Joys of SF: Essays in science and technology studies*. New York, NY: Open Court Press.

Levina, Marina. (2009). Regulation and discipline in the genomic age: A consideration of differences between genetic engineering and genomics. In Sam Binkley & Joe Capetillo (Eds.), *A Foucault for the 21st century: Governmentality, biopolitics and discipline in the new millennium* (pp. 308–319). Newcastle, England: Cambridge Scholars Publishing.

Levina, Marina. (2012). Our data, ourselves: Feminist narratives of empowerment in health 2.0 discourse. In Radhika Gajjala & Yeon Ju Oh (Eds.), *Cyberfeminism 2.0* (pp. 13–28). New York, NY: Peter Lang.

Levina, Marina, & Bui, Diem-my (Eds.). (2013). *Monster culture in the 21st century: A reader*. New York, NY: Bloomsbury.

Levina, Marina, & Kien, Grant. (2010). *Post-global network and everyday life*. New York, NY: Lang.

Lewton, Val (Producer), & Tourneur, Jacques (Director). (1943). *I walked with a zombie* [Motion picture]. United States: RKO Radio Pictures.

Li, Jiwei & Cardie, Claire. (2013, October 9). Twitter data stream used to predict flu outbreaks. *MIT Technology Review*. Retrieved from http://www.technologyreview.com/view/520116/twitter-datastream-used-to-predict-flu-outbreaks/

Linke, Uli. (1999). *Blood and nation: The European aesthetics of race*. Philadelphia, PA: University of Pennsylvania Press.

Loudermilk, A. (2003). Eating 'dawn' in the dark: Zombie desire and commodified identity in George A. Romero's 'Dawn of the dead.' *Journal of Consumer Culture*, *3*, 83–108.

Lupton, Deborah. (2013). Digitized health promotion: Personal responsibility for health in the Web 2.0 era. *The Sydney Health & Society Group*, 5, 1–22.

Macdonald, Andrew (Producer), & Boyle, Danny (Director). (2002). *28 days later* [Motion picture]. United Kingdom: 20th Century Fox.

Madrigal, Alexis. (2009, September 1). iPhone app finds disease outbreaks near you. *Wired*. Retrieved from http://www.wired.com/wiredscience/2009/09/outbreaksnearme/

Mantz, Jeffrey. (2013). On the frontlines of the zombie war in the Congo: Digital technology, the trade in conflict, minerals, and zombification. In Marina Levina & Diem-My Bui (Eds.), *Monster culture in the 21st century: A reader*. New York, NY: Bloomsbury.

Marcus, Mary. (2009, November 25). Mobile app helps people track H1N1, prevent flu. *USA Today*. Retrieved from http://usatoday30.usatoday.com/news/health/2009-11-25-new_flu-apps23_ST_N.htm

Marsh, Wendell, & McCune, Greg. (2011, May 19). CDC "Zombie Apocalypse" disaster campaign crashes website. *Reuters*. Retrieved from http://www.reuters.com/article/2011/05/19/us-zombies-idUSTRE74I7H420110519

Martin, Andrew, & Krauss, Clifford. (2009, April 28). Pork industry fights concerns over swine flu. *The New York Times*. Retrieved from http://www.nytimes.com/2009/04/29/business/economy/29trade.html

Marvin, Carolyn, & Ingle, David W. (1999). *Blood sacrifice and the nation: Totem rituals and the American flag*. Cambridge: Cambridge University Press.

Massumi, Brian. (2010). The future birth of the affective fact: The political ontology of threat. In Melissa Gregg & Gregory Seigworth (Eds.), *The affect theory reader* (pp. 52–71). Durham, NC: Duke University Press.

Mcgeary, Johanna. (2001, February 12). Death stalks a continent. *Time*, *157*(6).

McNeil, Donald G. (2012, May 7). A regime's tight grip on AIDS. *The New York Times*. Retrieved from http://www.nytimes.com/2012/05/08/health/a-regimes-tight-grip-lessons-from-cuba-in-aids-control.html

McRobbie, Angela, & Thornton, Sarah L. (1995). Rethinking moral panic for multi-mediated social worlds. *British Journal of Sociology* 46(4): 559–574.

Melton, John Gordon. (1994). *The vampire book: Encyclopedia of the undead*. Canton, MI: Visible Ink Press.

Michael, Mike, & Rosengarten, Marsha. (2012). HIV, Globalization and topology: Of prepositions and propositions. *Theory, Culture & Society* 29(4–5): 93–115.

Miller, Richard Lawrence. (1995). *Nazi justiz*. Westport: Praeger.

Mueller, Kristen. (2011). Nightmare of exploding pandemic. *Science*. Retrieved from http://www.sciencemag.org/content/334/6059/1064.1.full

Nelkin, Dorothy. (1999). Cultural perspectives on blood. In Eric A. Feldman & Robert Bayer (Eds.), *Blood feuds: AIDS, blood, and the politics of medical disaster* (pp. 273–292). New York, NY: Oxford University Press.

Nixon, Nicola. (1997). When Hollywood sucks, or, hungry girls, lost boys, and vampirism in the age of Reagan. In Joan Gordon, Veronica Hollinger, & Brian Aldiss (Eds.), *Blood read: The vampire as metaphor in contemporary culture* (pp. 115–128). Philadelphia, PA: University of Pennsylvania Press.

Paffenroth, Kim. (2006). *Gospel of the living dead: George Romero's visions of hell on earth*. Waco, TX: Baylor University Press.

Pandemic. (2006, November 7). *BBC News*. Retrieved from http://www.bbc.co.uk/sn/tvradio/programmes/horizon/broadband/tx/pandemic/

Paré, Ambroise. (1982). *On monsters and marvels*. (Janet L. Pallister, Trans.). Chicago, IL: The University of Chicago Press. (Original work published 1840)

Patton, Cindy. (2011). Pandemic, empire and the permanent state of exception. *Economic & Political Weekly*, 46(13), 103–110.

Pilkington, Ed. (2009, April 28). What's in a name? Governments debate 'swine flu' versus "Mexican' flu. *The Guardian*. Retrieved from http://www.theguardian.com/world/2009/apr/28/mexican-swine-flu-pork-name

Potter, Barr (Producer), & Carpenter, John (Director). (1998). *John Carpenter's vampires*. [Motion Picture]. United States: Columbia Pictures.

Riccardo, Martin. (1994). Living vampires, magic, and psychic attack. In Rosemary Ellen Guiley & J. B. Macabre (Eds.), *The complete vampire companion*. New York, NY: Macmillan.

Rohter, Larry. (2005, July 24). Prostitution puts U.S. and Brazil at odds on AIDS policy. *The New York Times*. Retrieved from http://www.nytimes.com/2005/07/24/international/americas/24brazil.html?pagewanted=all

Rose, Nikolas, & Novas, Carlos. (2005). Biological citizenship. In Aihwa Ong & Stephen J. Collier (Eds.), *Global assemblages: Technology, politics and ethics as anthropological problems*. New York, NY: Blackwell.

Rose, Nikolas. (2006). *The politics of life itself: Biomedicine, power, and subjectivity in the twenty-first century*, Princeton, NJ: Princeton University Press.

Rich, Emma, & Miah, Andy. (2009). Prosthetic surveillance: The medical governance of healthy bodies in cyberspace. *Surveillance & Society* 6(2): 163–177.

Ruane, Michael. (2009, September 2). Agencies worldwide use web to encourage citizens to do their own flu tracking. *The Washington Post*. Retrieved from http://www.washingtonpost.com/wp-dyn/content/article/2009/09/01/AR2009090103809.html

Sacks, Valerie. (1996). Women and AIDS: An analysis of media misrepresentations. *Social Science & Medicine*, 42(1), 59–73.

Saks, Eva. (1989). Representing miscegenation law. *Raritan*, 8(2), 29–41.

Salathe, Marcel, Linus Bengtsson, Todd J. Bodnar, Devon D. Brewer, John S. Brownstein, Caroline Buckee, Ellsworth M. Campbell et al. (2012). Digital epidemiology. *PLoS computational biology* 8, no. 7.

Salehi, Roxana, & Ali, S. Harris. (2006). The social and political context of disease outbreaks: The case of SARS in Toronto. *Canadian Public Policy 32*(4): 373–385.

Sandell, Rickard. (2006). *Pandemics: A security risk*. Madrid: Real Instituto Elcano.

Saunders, Robert. (2012). Undead spaces: Fear, globalisation, and the popular geopolitics of zombieism. *Geopolitics, 17*(1), 80–104.

Saussure, Ferdinand. (1998). *Course in general linguistics*. (Roy Harris, Trans.). Chicago, IL: Open Court. (Original work published 1916)

Savidge, Martin. (2009, April 30). 'Swine Flu' name offends Jews and Muslims. *World Focus*. Retrieved from http://worldfocus.org/blog/2009/04/30/swine-flu-name-offends-jews-and-muslims/5187/

Scales-Trent, Judy. (2001). Racial purity laws in the United States and Nazi Germany: The targeting process. *Human Rights Quarterly*, *23*(2), 260–307.

Scheper-Hughes, Nancy. (1992). *Death without weeping: The violence of everyday life in Brazil*. Berkeley, CA: University of California Press.

Scheper-Hughes, Nancy. (1993). AIDS, public health and human rights in Cuba. *Anthropology News*, *34*(7), 46–48.

Schillmeier, Michael. (2008). Globalizing risks: The cosmo-politics of SARS and its impact on globalizing sociology. *Mobilities*, 3(2), 179–199.

Schopp, Andrew. (1997). Cruising the alternative: Homoeroticism and the contemporary vampire. *Journal of Popular Culture* 30(4): 231–243.

Scott, Elaine, Slan, Jon (Producers), & Wu, David (Director). (2005). *Plague city: SARS in Toronto* [Motion picture]. Canada: Anchor Bay Entertainment.

Shah, Sonia. (2011). Viral disaster movie. *The Lancet*, 378(9798), 1211. Retrieved from http://www.thelancet.com/journals/lancet/article/PIIS0140-6736(11)61528-6/fulltext

Sharma, Sarah. (2009). Baring life and lifestyle in the non-place. *Cultural Studies*, *23*(1), 129–148.

Sheth, Amit. (2009). Citizen sensing, social signals, and enriching human experience. *IEEE Internet Computing*, *13*(4), 87–92.

Shildrick, Margrit. (2002). *Embodying the monster: Encounters with the vulnerable self*. London: Sage Publications.

Shilts, Randy. (1988). *And the band played on*. New York, NY: Penguin.

Siegel, Don (Director). (1956). *Invasion of the body snatchers* [Motion picture]. United States: Allied Artists Picture Corporation.

Simone, Renata (Director). (2007). "The age of AIDS" [Documentary]. United States: PBS.

Simone, Renata (Writer, Director). (2012). "Endgame" [Television series episode]. In David Fanning, Jacquie Jones & Michael Sullivan (Producers), *Frontline*. United States: PBS.

Slackman, Michael. (2009, May 24). Cleaning Cairo, but taking a livelihood. *The New York Times*. Retrieved from http://www.nytimes.com/2009/05/25/world/middleeast/25oink.html

Sontag, Susan. (1989). *Illness as metaphor and AIDS and its metaphors*. New York, NY: Doubleday.

Specter, Michael. (2005, February 28). Nature's bioterrorist: Is there any way to prevent a deadly avian-flu pandemic? *The New Yorker*. Retrieved from http://www.newyorker.com/archive/2005/02/28/050228fa_fact_specter

Stabile, Carol. A. (2001). Conspiracy or consensus? Reconsidering the moral panic. *Journal of Communication Inquiry*, *25*(3), 258–278. Retrieved from http://jci.sagepub.com/content/25/3/258

Stadler, Jonathan. (2003). Rumor, gossip and blame: Implications for HIV/AIDS prevention in the South African Lowveld. *AIDS Education and Prevention*, *15*(4), 357–368.

Starr, Douglas. (1998). *Blood: An epic history of medicine and commerce*. New York, NY: Quill.

Starr, Douglas. (2002, July 20). Bad blood: The 9/11 blood-donation disaster. *The New Republic*.

Starr, Douglas. P. (Writer), Marengo, Alex, Read, Nick, & Guercio, Gino Del (Directors). (2002). *Red gold* [Documentary]. In Alex Marengo, Nick Read, & Gino Del Guercio (Producers). United States: Films for the Humanities & Sciences.

Stengers, Isabelle. (2002). *Penser avec Whitehead*. Paris: Seuil.

Stern, Cori, Stern, Nicolas, Webb, Laurie (Producers), & Levine, Jonathan (Director). (2013). *Warm bodies* [Motion Picture]. United States: Lionsgate.

Stoker, Bram. *Dracula*. New York, NY: Broadview Press, 1997.

Stratton, Jon. (2011). Zombie trouble: Zombie texts, bare life and displaced people. *European Journal of Cultural Studies*, *14*(3), 265–281.

Surowiecki, James. (2003, May 12). The high cost of illness. *The New Yorker*. Retrieved from http://www.newyorker.com/archive/2003/05/12/030512ta_talk_surowiecki

Swanson, Janice, Gill, Ayesha, Wald, Karen, & Swanson, Karen. (1995). Comprehensive care and the sanatoria: Cuba's response to HIV/AIDS. *Journal of the Association of Nurses in AIDS Care*, *6*, 33–41.

Tapper, Melbourne. (1999). *In the blood: Sickle cell anemia and the politics of race*. Philadelphia, PA: University of Pennsylvania Press.

Taubin, Amy. (1995). Bloody tales. *Sight and Sound*, *5*(2), 8–11.

Terranova, Tiziana. (2004). *Network culture: Politics for the information*. London: Pluto Press.

Terry, Jennifer, & Urla, Jacqueline (Eds.). (1995). *Deviant bodies: Critical perspectives on difference in science and popular culture*. Bloomington, IN: Indiana University Press.

Thacker, Eugene. (2011). Necrologies; or, the death of the body politic. In Clough, Patricia Ticineto & Willse, Craig (Eds.), *Beyond biopolitics: Essays on the governance of life and death* (pp. 139–162). Durham, NC: Duke University Press.

Thompson, Kenneth. (1998). *Moral panics*. London: Routledge.

Tierney, John. (1990, October 19). AIDS in Africa: Experts study role of promiscuous sex in the epidemic. *The New York Times*. Retrieved from http://www.nytimes.com/1990/10/19/world/aids-in-africa-experts-study-role-of-promiscuous-sex-in-the-epidemic.html

Titmuss, Richard M. (1971). *The gift relationship: From human blood to social policy*. New York, NY: Pantheon.

Treichler, Paula A. (1999). *How to have theory in an epidemic: Cultural chronicles of AIDS*. Durham, NC: Duke University Press.

Trimble, Sarah. (2010). (White) rage: Affect, neoliberalism, and the family in *28 days Later* and *28 weeks later*. *The Review of Education, Pedagogy, and Cultural Studies*, *32*(3), 295–322.

U.S. Department of Health and Human Services, Centers for Disease Control and Prevention. (2012, July 16). Preparedness 101: Zombie pandemic. *Centers for Disease Control and Prevention*. Retrieved from http://www.cdc.gov/phpr/zombies_novella.htm

Ungar, Sheldon. (2001). Moral panic versus the risk society: The implications of the changing sites of social anxiety. *British Journal of Sociology*, *52*(2), 271–291.

Van Loon, Joost. (2000). Virtual risks in an age of cybernetic reproduction. In Barbara Adam, Ulrich Beck, & Joost Van Loon (Eds.), *The risk society and beyond: Critical issues for social theory* (pp. 165–182). London: Sage.

Vilsack, Tom. (2009). Statement from agricultural secretary Vilsack regarding animal health and 2009 pandemic H1N1 influenza. *USDA*. Retrieved from http://www.usda.gov/wps/portal/usda/usdahome?contentidonly=true&contentid=2009/09/0433.xml

Vint, Sherryl. (2013). Abject posthumanism: Neoliberalism, biopolitics and zombies. In Marina Levina & Diem-My Bui (Eds.), *Monster culture in the 21st century: A reader* (pp. 133–146). New York, NY: Bloomsbury.

Wailoo, Keith. (1997). *Drawing blood: Technology and disease identity in twentieth-century America*. Baltimore, MD: The Johns Hopkins University Press.

Wailoo, Keith. (2001) *Dying in the city of the blues: sickle cell anemia and the politics of race and health*. Durham, NC: The University of North Carolina Press Books.

Wald, Priscilla. (2008). *Contagious: Cultures, carriers, and the outbreak narrative*. Durham, NC: Duke University Press.

Wallis, Claudia. (1985, August 12). AIDS: A growing threat. *Time*, *126*(6).

Wallis, Patrick, & Nerlich, Brigette. (2005). Disease metaphors in new epidemics: The UK media framing of the 2003 SARS epidemic. *Social Science & Medicine*, 60(11), 2629–2639.

Watney, Simon. (1987). The spectacle of AIDS. *October*, *43*, 71–86. Retrieved from http://www.jstor.org/stable/3397565

Watney, Simon. (1988). *Policing desire: Pornography, AIDS, and the media*. Minneapolis, MN: University of Minnesota Press.

Webb, Jen, & Byrnand, Sam. (2008). Some kind of virus: The zombie as body and as trope. *Body & Society*, *14*(2), 83–98. Retrieved from http://dx.doi.org/10.1177/1357034X08090699

Weeks, Jeffrey. (1995). The body and sexuality. In Stuart Hall, David Held, Don Hubert & Kenneth Thompson (Eds.), *Modernity: An introduction to modern society* (pp. 363–395). Cambridge, UK: Polity Press.

Weston, Kath. (2001). Kinship, controversy, and the sharing of substance: The race/class politics of blood transfusion. In Sarah Franklin & Susan McKinnon (Eds.), *Relative values: Reconfiguring kinship studies* (pp. 147–174). Durham, NC: Duke University Press.

White, Luise. (1993). Cars out of place: Vampires, technology and labor in eastern and central Africa. *Representations*, *43*, 27–50.

Will, George. (2000, January 17). AIDS crushes a continent. *Newsweek*, *135*(3).

Wolf, Leonard. (1997). *Dracula: The connoisseur's guide*. New York, NY: Broadway.

Wood, Robin. (1996). Burying the undead: The use and obsolescence of Count Dracula. In Barry Keith Grant (Ed.), *The dread of difference* (pp. 308–319). Austin, TX: University of Texas Press.

Woolf, Aviva. (2013, October 9). Site uses social media to track illness. *Phys.org*. http://phys.org/news/2013-10-site-social-media-track-illness.html.

Youde, Jeremy. (2012). Biosurveillance, human rights, and the zombie plague. *Global Change, Peace & Security: formerly Pacifica Review: Peace, Security & Global Change*, *24*(1), 83–93. Retrieved from http://dx.doi.org/10.1080/14781158.2012.641278

Zanger, Jules. (1997). Metaphor into metonymy: The vampire next door. In Gordon, Joan, Hollinger, Veronica, & Aldiss, Brian (Eds.), *Blood read: The vampire as metaphor in contemporary culture* (pp. 17–26). Philadelphia, PA: University of Pennsylvania Press.

Zoler, Mitchel L. (2013, March 25). Flu Near You spearheads U.S. participatory surveillance growth. *Family Practice News*. Retrieved from http://www.familypracticenews.com/index.php?id=2934&type=98&tx_ttnews[tt_news]=141801&cHash=da03e20e36

INDEX

C

D

E

F

G

H

S

T

V

W

Z

Global Crises and the Media

Simon Cottle, *General Editor*

From climate change to the war on terror, financial meltdowns to forced migrations, pandemics to world poverty, and humanitarian disasters to the denial of human rights, these and other crises represent the dark side of our globalized planet. They are endemic to the contemporary global world and so too are they highly dependent on the world's media.

Each of the specially commissioned books in the *Global Crises and the Media* series examines the media's role, representation, and responsibility in covering major global crises. They show how the media can enter into their constitution, enacting them on the public stage and thereby helping to shape their future trajectory around the world. Each book provides a sophisticated and empirically engaged understanding of the topic in order to invigorate the wider academic study and public debate about the most pressing and historically unprecedented global crises of our time.

For further information about the series and submitting manuscripts, please contact:

Dr. Simon Cottle
Cardiff School of Journalism
Cardiff University, Room 1.28
The Bute Building, King Edward VII Ave.
Cardiff CF10 3NB
United Kingdom
CottleS@cardiff.ac.uk

To order other books in this series, please contact our Customer Service Department at:

(800) 770-LANG (within the U.S.)
(212) 647-7706 (outside the U.S.)
(212) 647-7707 FAX

Or browse online by series at:

www.peterlang.com

www.ingramcontent.com/pod-product-compliance
Ingram Content Group UK Ltd.
Pitfield, Milton Keynes, MK11 3LW, UK
UKHW021839100926
8556IPUK00004B/442

9 781433 115523